Immunology and Immune System Disorders

Celiac Disease

An Update

IMMUNOLOGY AND IMMUNE SYSTEM DISORDERS

Additional books in this series can be found on Nova's website under the Series tab.

Additional e-books in this series can be found on Nova's website under the e-book tab.

IMMUNOLOGY AND IMMUNE SYSTEM DISORDERS

CELIAC DISEASE

AN UPDATE

MAURO BOZZOLA
CRISTINA MEAZZA
GIUSEPPE MAGGIORE
AND
SILVIA NASTASIO

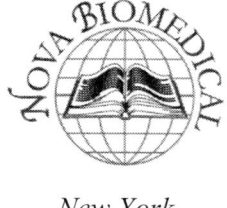

New York

Copyright © 2014 by Nova Science Publishers, Inc.

All rights reserved. No part of this book may be reproduced, stored in a retrieval system or transmitted in any form or by any means: electronic, electrostatic, magnetic, tape, mechanical photocopying, recording or otherwise without the written permission of the Publisher.

For permission to use material from this book please contact us:
Telephone 631-231-7269; Fax 631-231-8175
Web Site: http://www.novapublishers.com

NOTICE TO THE READER

The Publisher has taken reasonable care in the preparation of this book, but makes no expressed or implied warranty of any kind and assumes no responsibility for any errors or omissions. No liability is assumed for incidental or consequential damages in connection with or arising out of information contained in this book. The Publisher shall not be liable for any special, consequential, or exemplary damages resulting, in whole or in part, from the readers' use of, or reliance upon, this material. Any parts of this book based on government reports are so indicated and copyright is claimed for those parts to the extent applicable to compilations of such works.

Independent verification should be sought for any data, advice or recommendations contained in this book. In addition, no responsibility is assumed by the publisher for any injury and/or damage to persons or property arising from any methods, products, instructions, ideas or otherwise contained in this publication.

This publication is designed to provide accurate and authoritative information with regard to the subject matter covered herein. It is sold with the clear understanding that the Publisher is not engaged in rendering legal or any other professional services. If legal or any other expert assistance is required, the services of a competent person should be sought. FROM A DECLARATION OF PARTICIPANTS JOINTLY ADOPTED BY A COMMITTEE OF THE AMERICAN BAR ASSOCIATION AND A COMMITTEE OF PUBLISHERS.

Additional color graphics may be available in the e-book version of this book.

Library of Congress Cataloging-in-Publication Data

ISBN: 978-1-63117-088-1

Library of Congress Control Number: 2014933504

Published by Nova Science Publishers, Inc. † New York

Contents

Preface		vii
Acknowledgments		ix
Chapter 1	Spectrum of Gluten Intolerance: From Celiac Disease to "Non-Celiac" Gluten Sensitivity *Silvia Nastasio and Giuseppe Maggiore*	1
Chapter 2	Diagnostic Approach to Short Stature in Children with Celiac Disease *Cristina Meazza and Mauro Bozzola*	49
Index		77

PREFACE

While the interest in celiac disease outside of Europe can be considered relatively recent and booming fast, especially in North America where an astonishingly sharp increase in followers of a gluten-free diet is seen, Italian physicians and scientists have been familiar with this condition for a long time. Indeed, the contributions made by Italian investigators to the advancement of our knowledge in celiac disease have been cutting-edge and outstanding in many regards: unraveling many patho-physiological aspects, detecting the ever-evolving spectrum of clinical manifestations, redefining its diagnostic guidelines.

It is therefore no surprise that this agile book on celiac disease is authored by my colleagues and friends Prof. Bozzola and Prof. Maggiore.

A thorough and critical update on the current knowledge on this unique autoimmune disease (exploring all of its many facets) is presented in a rigorous yet accessible style that is sure to meet the favor of residents and fellows alike. The booklet also includes a special focus on the frequently encountered and often puzzling problem of short stature (or stunted height gain) in the context of celiac disease. In fact, 15% of the almost 1,000 children in our Chicago Celiac Disease Center came to be diagnosed on the basis of failure to proper gain height, but in only half of them, was celiac disease the direct culprit. A clinically sound, effective approach to this problem is laid out, which will greatly benefit pediatricians and endocrinologists dealing with these children and often facing the dilemma of whether or not to start a treatment with GH.

Thus, I am particularly happy to welcome this Italian-generated booklet in the family of the most updated, reliable educational tools available on our fascinating celiac disease, and am sure it will encounter the success it deserves in the wider online community!

Chicago, IL January 13, 2014

Stefano Guandalini, M.D.
Professor of Pediatrics
Founder and Medical Director of the University
of Chicago Celiac Disease Center
Past President of the North American Society
for the Study of Celiac Disease

ACKNOWLEDGMENTS

The authors are grateful to Ms. Laurene Kelly for the English revision of the manuscript.

In: Celiac Disease: An Update
Editors: M. Bozzola, C. Meazza et al.
ISBN: 978-1-63117-088-1
© 2014 Nova Science Publishers, Inc.

Chapter 1

SPECTRUM OF GLUTEN INTOLERANCE: FROM CELIAC DISEASE TO "NON-CELIAC" GLUTEN SENSITIVITY

Silvia Nastasio, M.D.[*], and Giuseppe Maggiore, M.D.[†]
[1]Clinical and Experimental Medicine Department, Pediatric Gastroenterology, University of Pisa, Pisa, Italy

ABSTRACT

Celiac disease (CD) is a systemic immune-mediated disorder triggered by dietary gluten in genetically susceptible persons. CD affects about 1% of the population in Europe and North-America, however there are significant differences in neighboring countries. Since the late '80s the epidemiology of CD has been depicted as an iceberg where its visible peak represents patients with different clinical manifestations, while its submerged part represents those with very minimal or no symptoms at all. Treatment consists of a gluten-free diet (GFD).

Celiac disease is a multifactorial disease in which genetic predisposition and environmental factors contribute to onset of the disease. The principal determinants of genetic susceptibility to CD are the major histocompatibility class II HLA molecules. Specifically, the HLA-DQ2 haplotype is expressed in the majority of patients with CD (90%),

---

[*] E-mail: silvia.nastasio@gmail.com.
[†] E-mail: giuseppe.maggiore@med.unipi.it.

whereas the HLA-DQ8 haplotype is expressed only in 5% of patients. The remaining 5% of patients have at least one of the two genes encoding DQ2 (DQB1*0201 or DQA1*0501).

Celiac disease presents with a broad spectrum of signs and symptoms depending on age, individual sensitivity to gluten and on the amount of toxic proteins ingested with the diet. Malabsorption syndrome with growth failure, malnutrition, chronic diarrhea, steatorrhea, edema (secondary to hypoalbuminemia), abdominal distension and muscle wasting are all characteristics that historically identify this disease. However, over time numerous different presentations of CD have been described.

Diagnosis of CD is based on serological testing by specific markers, and by histological analysis of duodenal biopsies. Young patients with CD should be monitored regularly for normal growth and development, appearance of symptoms, and adherence to GFD. Monitoring adherence to GFD should be based on a combination of personal and dietetic history and serological testing. A diagnosis of non-celiac gluten sensitivity should be considered only when CD has been excluded by appropriate testing.

INTRODUCTION

The spectrum of disorders related to gluten ingestion in humans includes, an allergic condition (*wheat allergy*), a condition due to genetic and autoimmune factors (*celiac disease*) and a recently described and controversial form defined as *"non-celiac gluten sensitivity"*. In this chapter celiac disease will be discussed in detail. It is indeed the most clinically relevant condition in which genetic predisposition and environmental factors interact to trigger an autoimmune response, and is the only human condition in which the causative antigen is known. Gluten allergy and the so-called *non-celiac gluten sensitivity* will also be briefly described.

CELIAC DISEASE

Celiac disease (CD) is a systemic immune-mediated disorder triggered by dietary gluten in genetically susceptible persons [1]. Treatment of CD consists of a gluten-free diet (GFD) which determines remission of intestinal damage; it protects against the risk of developing autoimmune diseases associated with CD and "normalizes" the mortality risk related to the disease itself. Mortality in the celiac patient is indeed significantly higher than in non-celiac patients if gluten is not excluded from the diet and it depends mainly on the increased risk of developing T-cell lymphomas and non-Hodgkin's lymphomas.

History of Celiac Disease

Bread was already known in ancient Egypt where bread was not only considered a dietary staple, but was also considered currency for trade in everyday life.

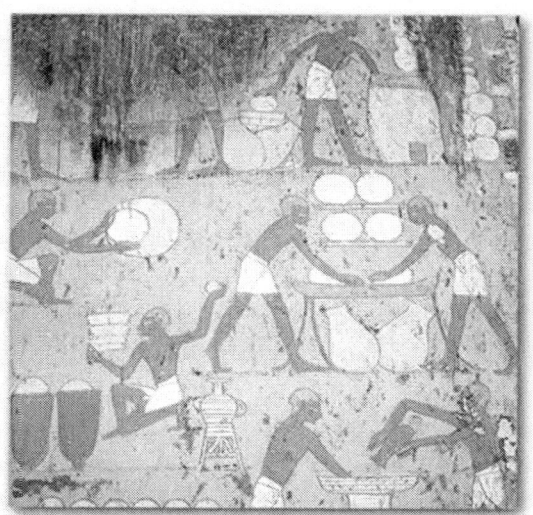
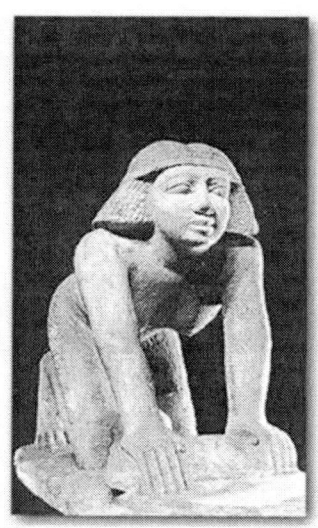

Although typical CD symptoms and clinical signs, namely those related to enteropathy were first described in the third century b.C. in the "celiac diathesis" description of an adult by *Aretaeus of Cappadocia*, the link between the clinical disease manifestations and exposure to a food stuff was only recognized at the end of the nineteenth century by a British pediatrician, Samuel Jones Gee, who was working in London at the Hospital for Sick Children, Great Hormond Street; he claimed that "if the patient can be cured at all, it must be by means of diet". However, it was only in 1940 that a pediatrician from the Netherlands, Willem-Karel Dicke, recognized wheat flour, as the cause of CD [2].

The first scientific consensus document on CD, followed the Interlaken meeting of the European Society of Pediatric Gastroenterology and Nutrition (ESPGAN) in 1969, and was published in the Journal of Acta Paediatrica in 1970 [3]. In this document CD was defined as a permanent condition of gluten intolerance characterized by abnormal morphology of the small intestinal mucosa, its normalization on gluten withdrawal, and the relapse on reintroduction of gluten.

In order to meet the aforementioned criteria, the diagnostic sequence proposed by ESPGAN, therefore required, at least three biopsies of the small intestine: the first biopsy during an unrestricted diet in order to demonstrate the enteropathy, a second biopsy after a period of GFD, to demonstrate *restitutio ad integrum* of the mucosa and the third, after a period of gluten challenge to document the possible recurrence of mucosal damage. This sequence of small bowel biopsies was a means of differentiating CD from other, transient, causes of abnormal small intestinal mucosa by proving, at the time of challenge, the long lasting sensitivity to gluten. A critical review of these criteria after less than 10 years (1978) showed, however, that "only" two-thirds of the ESPGAN members strictly agreed with these diagnostic criteria, especially regarding the need for a third biopsy; however, the Interlaken criteria were not modified [4]. The introduction of new diagnostic tools (anti-gliadin, anti-reticulin, and later anti-endomysium antibodies) and the increased awareness of the great mucosal sensitivity to gluten variability, stimulated an ESPGAN "*ad hoc*" workshop in Budapest in 1989. The conclusions of this workshop were published in 1990 [5]; it was established, for the first time, that a challenge with gluten (and therefore the third biopsy) was not mandatory to diagnose CD. Furthermore the discretionary use of the second biopsy for the demonstration of mucosal damage normalization after a GFD was established. On the other hand, a gluten challenge was suggested in case of doubts about the initial diagnosis and lack of adequacy of the clinical response to a GFD.

In conclusion, in this document it was stated that the diagnosis of CD does not require further confirmation if the initial diagnosis is based firstly on the appearance of flat small intestinal mucosa with the histological features of hyperplastic crypts and villous atrophy while the patient is consuming adequate amounts of gluten, and secondly an unequivocal and full clinical remission after withdrawal of gluten from the diet.

Also, it was affirmed for the first time how the finding of circulating antibodies (IgA anti-gliadin, anti-reticulin, and anti-endomysiun) at the time of diagnosis and their disappearance when the patient was on a GFD added weight to the diagnosis.

In the last ten years we have been confronted with an "explosion" of knowledge regarding CD that has led to the recent publication of new consensus documents and updated guidelines. The most relevant documents are the new ESPGHAN guidelines published in 2012 [6], the guidelines of the World Gastroenterology Organization [7] and the review of the terminology regarding the different forms of CD, completed by an international task force of experts and published at the beginning of 2013 [8].

The main conclusions of the new ESPGHAN guidelines are as follows:

- CD diagnosis depends on gluten-dependent symptoms, CD-specific antibody levels, the presence of HLA-DQ2 and/or HLA-DQ8, and characteristic histological changes (villous atrophy and crypt hyperplasia) in the duodenal biopsy.
- high TG2-antibody levels (10 times ULN for a standard curve-based calculation) as measured by a qualified laboratory in a symptomatic patient has such high diagnostic accuracy that omitting the duodenal biopsy might be possible.
- CD diagnosis should be confirmed by an antibody decline and a clinical response to a GFD.
- gluten challenge and repetitive biopsies will be necessary only in selected patients in whom diagnostic uncertainty persists.

Gluten

Gluten is a protein complex found in wheat, rye, barley, oats or their crossbred varieties and derivatives thereof. This complex consists mostly of prolamins, a group of peptides soluble in alcohol, which account for about half of the proteins of ripe wheat. The term gluten refers especially to a group of prolamins of wheat (gliadin and glutenin) although other prolamins antigenically similar are found in rye (secalin) and barley (hordein). Maize prolamins, because of a different phylogenetic evolution, do not cause damage in the celiac patient and likely oat prolamins do not either. A GFD indicates a diet free from wheat, barley and rye as well as from other cereals such as triticale, kamut and spelt.

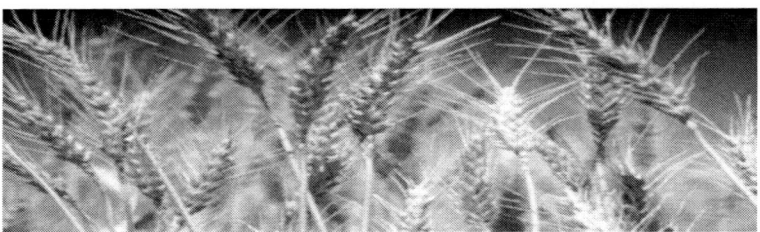

Gluten is poorly digested in the human intestine, irrespective of the presence or absence of CD. Its oligopeptides cross the intestinal mucosa intact reaching the submucosa where they are deamidated by tissue transglutaminase type 2 (tTG2). This process of deamidation favors high affinity binding with the HLA-DQ2 and DQ8 molecules expressed on the surface of T lymphocytes and, in the celiac patient, trigger an inflammatory and immune-mediated response typical of the disease. Alimentary gluten content is measured by enzyme immunoassay and is regulated by the Codex Alimentarius which defines gluten-free foods as those foods whose gluten content is <20 mg/kg.

Epidemiology

Celiac disease affects about 1% of the population in Europe and North-America, with significant differences in neighboring countries (from 0.3% in Germany to 2.4% in Finland). Celiac disease is also diagnosed in Australia, New Zealand and South America, especially in individuals of European descent, but it is also recognized with increasing frequency in different geographic areas such as the Middle East, Indian Ocean, China and North Africa, with a particularly high peak prevalence in indigenous populations, such as 5.6% in the Saharawi population (Western Sahara) [9]. Factors responsible for this increase in new cases of CD in developing countries, include westernization of the local diet, changes in wheat production and preparation, increased awareness of the disease and simplified diagnostic techniques.

The estimated CD prevalence in Italy is 0.7%, but the number of patients currently undiagnosed is thought to be largely superior to known cases. This phenomenon is related to the presence of prevalent forms of CD with nonspecific symptoms. In Italy therefore, about 100,000 people have been diagnosed with CD, but it is believed that there are at least another 500,000 undiagnosed cases.

Since the late '80s the epidemiology of CD has been represented by an iceberg (figure 1). Its visible peak represents patients with different clinical manifestations of CD, and its submerged part represents those who show very minimal or no symptoms at all.

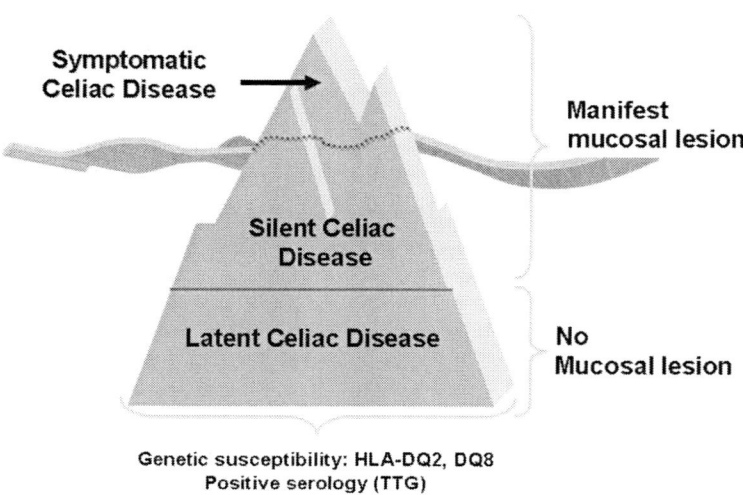

Figure 1. The celiac iceberg.

The introduction of a simple screening test facilitated the redefinition of CD distribution, and highlighted the fact that CD is a rather frequent condition, although with a polymorphous clinical spectrum, in which gastrointestinal manifestations may be marginal or even absent. A "new view" of CD has been adopted, thanks to the use of serological tests, which have enabled the development of screening programs in different parts of the world.

The prevalence of CD is moderately higher in women than in men (from 1.5 to 2 times), and it is significantly higher in first-degree relatives of celiac patients (10-15%), in patients with acquired endocrine disorders such as diabetes mellitus type 1 (T1DM) (3-16%), Hashimoto's thyroiditis (5%), in those with hepatobiliary disease (4-16%) and in patients with other conditions such as IgA deficiency (9%). Furthermore, there s a number of genetic disorders in which CD association is significantly higher than expected, such as Down syndrome (5%), Turner syndrome (3%) and Williams syndrome.

Genetic Factor Influence

Celiac disease is a multifactorial disease in which genetic predisposition, along with environmental factors, contributes to the onset of the disease [10]. The high incidence of CD in first-degree relatives of celiac patients and high concordance in monozygotic twins (80%) suggests a strong genetic component. It can therefore be assumed that the "celiac constitution" is written in the genome, while the environment (age of weaning with gluten introduction, gluten intake, gastrointestinal infections, allergies) intervenes "modulating" the expression of the disease. The principal determinants of genetic susceptibility to CD are the major histocompatibility class II HLA molecules (*HLA-Human Leukocyte Antigen Complex*). Specifically, development of CD class II HLA DQ2 (DQA1*05-DQB1*02) and/or DQ8 (DQA1*03-DQB1*0302), which are glycoproteins expressed on the cell membrane and encoded by the genes HLA-DQA1 and HLA-DQB1 gene located on chromosome 6p21.3, are necessary for the development of CD. DQ2 and DQ8 haplotypes expressed on the surface of antigen-presenting cells can bind activated (deamidated) gluten peptides and trigger an abnormal immune response.

The immunocompetent cells of individuals carrying these haplotypes are in fact able to interact with "high affinity" specific epitopes of gliadin "activated" (i.e., deamidated) by transglutaminase in the submucosa of the small intestine, thus triggering an abnormal immune response. The recognition of the complex HLA-antigen by helper T lymphocytes of the intestinal mucosa consequently determines the subsequent release of pro-inflammatory cytokines responsible for the development of the duodenal mucosal lesion. The HLA-DQ2 haplotype is expressed in the majority of patients with CD (90%) whereas the HLA-DQ8 haplotype is expressed in only another 5% of patients. The remaining 5% of patients have at least one of the two genes encoding for DQ2 (DQB1*0201 or DQA1*0501).

Bound to HLA-DQ2 there is a strong gene dosage effect: homozygous individuals have a 5 fold higher risk of developing the disease compared to heterozygotes. In homozygotes, also the magnitude of the response to gluten is greater because, compared to heterozygous, they have a greater number of HLA-DQ2 molecules on the surface of antigen presenting cells that are able to bind with high affinity gluten peptides. In conclusion, the presence of the HLA haplotypes DQ2 and/or DQ8 is necessary for CD to develop, while the absence of these haplotypes has a high negative predictive value for the diagnosis of CD.

However, the DQ2 and DQ8 haplotypes are necessary but not sufficient for the development of CD. The HLA-DQ2 haplotype is indeed expressed in about 30-35% of the general population and in 60-70% of the people who have an affected first-degree relative. On the other hand, only 10% of people with this genetic predisposition develop CD. So far, at least 39 non-HLA genes that confer a predisposition to the disease have been identified, most of which are involved in inflammatory and immune responses.

At present, the concept of individual genetic risk for CD, should be restricted to relatives of individuals with CD presenting HLA DQ2 or DQ8. Such individuals have a risk of developing CD that is variable from 2 to 20%, depending on the degree of kinship and the number of copies of the HLA-DQ2 gene possessed.

Environmental Factor Influence

The main environmental factors that have an important role in the development of celiac disease are: breastfeeding and timing of gluten introduction at weaning. The introduction of gluten before 4 months of life is associated with an increased risk of developing the disease, while the introduction of gluten after 7 months of life results in a significant risk reduction.

In fact, it is rather the introduction of gluten during continued breastfeeding that seems to be associated with a significantly lower risk of developing CD. A further suggested trigger to the loss of gluten tolerance is intestinal infections, in particular those caused by rotavirus, although this assumption still remains controversial.

Pathogenesis

A peculiar feature of CD, as compared to other autoimmune diseases, is the evidence of an environmental trigger, gliadin. The primary manifestation is represented by histological damage to the mucosa of the duodenal tract, and by an immunological reaction of the lamina propria. The key agents of CD are immunogenic, glutamine containing gliadin peptides that are resistant to gastric and pancreatic enzyme digestion, which thus reach the lamina propria of the intestinal mucosa. This is achieved through modifications of intercellular junctions and increased intestinal permeability. Gliadin, in fact, causes the increased expression of zonulin (a molecule that regulates the polymerization of actin microfilaments and the opening of tight junctions) with a consequent increase in intestinal permeability and therefore facilitated entry of toxic and immunogenic peptides in the lamina propria. In the intestinal mucosa, tTG2 released in the extracellular compartment catalyzes the deamidation of gliadin peptides, creating immunostimulatory epitopes with a higher affinity for DQ2 and DQ8 molecules. The resulting modified peptides are presented in complex with HLA DQ2 or DQ8 by antigen presenting cells to T helper $CD4^+$ [11].

The recognition of the HLA-peptide complex by T lymphocytes determines their activation and the release of various cytokines including IL-15 and INF-γ. These molecules induce the activation and clonal expansion of B cells, which produce antibodies directed not only against gluten, but also autoantibodies against tTG2 itself. Other cytokines stimulate fibroblasts and inflammatory cells to secrete matrix metalloproteinases, with consequent tissue remodeling and further release of tTG2 in the extracellular compartment.

At the same time as activation of these mechanisms and the increase in infiltrating CD4$^+$T lymphocytes in the lamina propria, there is also an increase in intraepithelial lymphocytes which exert cytolytic activity and determine the damage of the epithelium. The lesions of the intestinal mucosa (villous atrophy and crypt hyperplasia) found on biopsy are the result of this immunological process, which is dynamic and adaptable over time.

Natural History

The production of tTG2 autoantibodies, in the mucosa of the small intestine, is the first in a series of events that leads to the development of CD. After the production of mucosal antibodies, there is a gradual increase of these autoantibodies in the serum without signs of enteropathy [12]. Only later does the enteropathy develop with the onset of symptoms and the possible development of complications. The duration of each of these phases varies from a few weeks to several years and these events are not all necessarily present in the same patient. Potential CD for example, is characterized by the presence of "celiac" autoantibodies in the serum of patients with normal gut mucosa morphology [13]. A variable degree of enteropathy develops over time in a subset of these patients. In contrast to the assumption that the enteropathy develops in early childhood, as a direct consequence of weaning and therefore is due to the exposure to gluten, more recent studies have shown that the conversion towards the development of an autoimmune response triggered by gluten can occur at any time of life, even with a long latency. Thus, genetic susceptibility and contact with gluten, while necessary, are not sufficient to develop gluten intolerance, and consequently CD. Finally, occasionally, lost tolerance to gluten may be regained, thus genetically predisposed individuals, with anti-tTG2, have been shown to reverse their serology and normalize the enteropathy, despite the persistence of exposure to gluten. This phenomenon, however sporadic, which does not affect the principle of persistent intolerance to gluten in the celiac patient, may vary over time.

A Polymorphic Clinical Picture

Celiac patients present with a broad spectrum of signs and symptoms which depend on age, individual sensitivity to gluten and amount of proteins ingested with the diet. Malabsorption syndrome with growth failure, malnutrition, chronic diarrhea, steatorrhea, edema (secondary to hypoalbuminemia), abdominal distension and muscle wasting should be considered when evaluating the clinical picture that historically identifies this disease (figure 2).

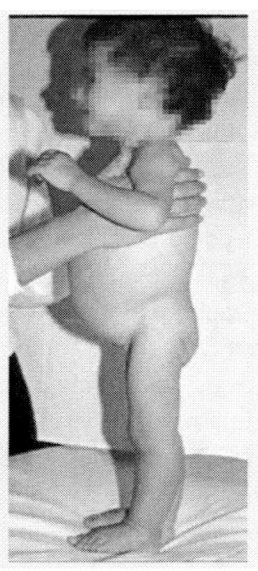

Figure 2. Classical CD in a child.

Over time numerous forms of CD have been described:

1. *Typical CD* has historically been described as a gluten-induced enteropathy presenting with signs or symptoms of malabsorption (such as diarrhea or malnutrition) or a malabsorption syndrome (indicated by weight loss, steatorrhoea and edema secondary to hypoalbuminemia). The use of this term is questionable in that the clinical presentation of CD has changed over time, and the word 'typical' implies that this form is the most frequently encountered

form of CD. In contrast, many current patients have symptoms such as anemia, fatigue and abdominal pain. Therefore the use of the term typical CD is discouraged [8].

2. *Classical CD* is an alternative for typical CD and is defined by the presence of a gluten-induced enteropathy presenting with signs and symptoms of malabsorption. While recognizing that these symptoms are not specific to CD, the use of the classical CD term, as defined above, has been encouraged, because the term 'classical' does not imply that this type of CD is more common than CD without clinical malabsorption. Children with classical CD present with typical malabsorption signs and symptoms such as failure to thrive, diarrhea, abdominal distension, muscle wasting, poor appetite and irritability [8]. Classical CD usually manifests between the age of 6 months and 2 years after gluten has been introduced to the diet. The so called "celiac crisis" defined by acute explosive watery diarrhea, marked abdominal distension, dehydratation, hypotension, lethargy, hypoproteinemia, and metabolic and electrolyte imbalances is now rarely observed.

3. *Atypical CD* has historically been used to describe patients with gluten-induced enteropathy presenting with non-specific gastrointestinal symptoms including symptoms suggestive of irritable bowel syndrome without evidence of malabsorption (weight loss) or with extraintestinal manifestations (table 1), such as iron and folic acid deficiency with or without anemia, dermatitis herpetiformis, delayed puberty, short stature, enamel defects (figure 3), recurrent aphthous stomatitis (figure 4). The use of this term is also discouraged [8].

4. *Asymptomatic or silent CD* identifies patients who do not manifest any symptoms commonly associated with CD. These patients are often diagnosed through testing of populations enrolled in screening programs or in case-finding strategies for detecting CD in patients with disorders that are associated with a high risk for CD. However, many of these patients who suffer from decreased quality of life and sometimes minor symptoms (eg, fatigue) are only recognized after the introduction of a GFD. These patients do not suffer from true asymptomatic CD and should be reclassified as having subclinical CD [8].

Table 1. Extraintestinal manifestations of CD

SKELETAL SYSTEM:
• Osteopenia/osteoporosis
• Arthritis
• Enamel defects
ENDOCRINE SYSTEM:
• Short stature
• Delayed puberty
• Infertility
CENTRAL NERVOUS SYSTEM:
• Epilepsy with occipital calcifications
• Depression
• Ataxia
OTHER SYSTEMS:
• Myelopathy
• Iron deficiency anemia refractory to oral iron supplementation
• Hypertransaminasemia
• Dermatitis herpetiformis

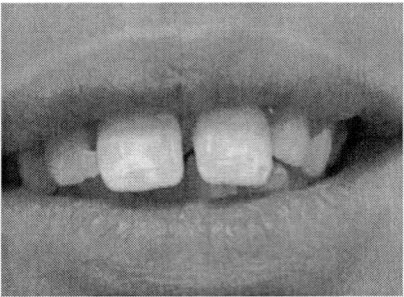

Figure 3. Enamel defects in a celiac patient.

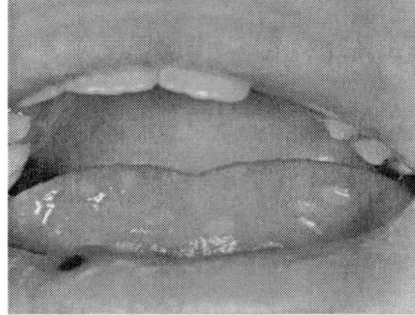

Figure 4. Aphthous stomatitis in a celiac patient.

5. *Latent CD* identifies patients with a positive CD serology, but with normal mucosa or absence of villous atrophy [8]. The term latent CD has also been discouraged.
6. *Potential CD* relates to people who are at increased risk of developing CD as indicated by a positive CD serology. Potential CD is also often used as a synonym for latent CD with inconsistent meanings. For some, potential CD means that the patient has a positive CD serology, but a normal small intestinal mucosa; for others, the intestinal mucosa might show an increased number of intraepithelial T lymphocytes (IELs) in the villi or an increased expression of the $\gamma\delta$ activation receptor. Treatment for potential CD is still controversial, as it is not clear whether a GFD is necessary. It is definitely important to monitor these patients over time in order to eventually start treating them before complications related to the disease appear.
7. *Refractory CD* consists of persistent or recurrent malabsorptive symptoms and signs with villous atrophy despite a strict GFD for more than 12 months in the absence of other causes of villous atrophy or malignant complications [8]. Refractory CD is defined as primary when there is no initial response to a GFD or as secondary if a relapse occurs following an initial response to a GFD.

It is critical to define whether the patient is really celiac or if there is another cause for the enteropathy and its symptoms, such as inadvertent or unintentional introduction of gluten with the diet or lymphoma. Refractory CD is especially rare in children; whereas in adult patients two different categories have been identified: type I, in which a normal IEL phenotype is found; and type II, in which there is a clonal expansion of an aberrant IEL population. The abnormal phenotype is supported by the loss of normal surface markers CD3, CD4 and CD8 with preserved expression of intracytoplasmic CD3 (CD3e) in >50% of IELs as evaluated by immunohistochemistry or >20% as determined by flow cytometry, and by the detection of a clonal rearrangement of T-cell receptor chains (γ or δ) by PCR.

The malabsorption syndrome with weight loss, chronic diarrhea, abdominal distension, must be regarded by far as the classical clinical picture of the disease, even though we now know that it is a relatively rare presentation. Celiac disease is indeed characterized by a large variety of gastrointestinal symptoms, even mild ones (abdominal pain, flatulence, dyspepsia), and in a large number of cases it is mainly characterized by extraintestinal manifestations.

Among these, isolated growth failure is frequent and it can be confused with a less common growth hormone deficiency.

In Table 2 the three main clinical expression groups for CD are summarized:

- The group with enteropathy and malabsorption is strictly gluten-associated, not necessarily accompanied by diarrhea, but with milder gastrointestinal symptoms and symptoms related to malabsorption (iron deficiency anemia, failure to thrive, and sometimes osteopenia);
- The group with an immune-mediated disease, includes a number of clinical conditions in which the association with gluten is extremely clear (dermatitis herpetiformis), and others which have only been occasionally described (alopecia, connectivitis, hemocytopenias, polyneuropathy) or suggested by the results of clinical and epidemiological studies (T1DM, autoimmune thyroid disease, autoimmune liver diseases).
- The group with associations between specific morbid conditions and CD, in particular Turner syndrome and Down syndrome, might be useful for the better understanding of a genetic regulation of CD.

It is particularly interesting that the extraintestinal manifestations of gluten intolerance (dermatitis herpetiformis, and even lymphoma) may also occur in the absence of intestinal mucosa subatrophy. Concerning non-Hodgkin's lymphoma of the gastrointestinal tract, and the risk of cancer in general, as early as 1989 it was suggested that there exists a causal relationship between onset of cancer (oral cavity, pharynx, esophagus) and duration of the diet. However, it was shown that in celiac patients on a

GFD for at least five years, this risk was not higher than that of the general population.

Table 2. Clinical expression of CD

Secondary to malabsorption	Secondary to mechanisms other than malabsorption * # ° (eg, autoimmunity)	Associations
- Iron deficiency anemia - Mixed normocytic anemia (lack of compensation between iron and folate) - Isolated growth failure - Osteopenia - Poliabortivity - Fatty liver - Abdominal pain / bloating	- Dermatitis herpetiformis* - Enamel Defect* - Ataxia gluten* - Alopecia* - Osteopenia# - Isolated hypertransaminasemia* - Insulin-dependent diabetes° - Autoimmune thyroid disease° - Autoimmune hepatitis° - Primary biliary cirrhosis - Inflammatory Bowel Disease - Sjögren's syndrome° - Addison's Disease° - Recurrent aphthous stomatitis# - Myasthenia gravis - Autoimmune atrophic gastritis - Recurrent Pericarditis# - Autoimmune hemocytopenias°# - Psoriasis°# - Polyneuropathy/myopathy°# - Epilepsy (with or without intracranial calcifications)* - Vasculitis# - Hypo/hyperparathyroidism# - Dilated cardiomyopathy - IgA deficiency#?	- Down Syndrome - Turner Syndrome - Williams Syndrome - Congenital heart disease - IgA deficiency

*Strictly dependent on gluten intake or #demonstrated in a variable number of cases.
°There are epidemiological data suggesting that gluten intolerance is not recognized and therefore not treated, favoring the onset of the disease. The symbol (?) indicates that it is uncertain in which categories IgA deficiency belongs to.

It is particularly interesting that the extraintestinal manifestations of gluten intolerance (dermatitis herpetiformis, and even lymphoma) may also occur in the absence of intestinal mucosa subatrophy. Concerning non-Hodgkin's lymphoma of the gastrointestinal tract, and the risk of cancer in general, as early as 1989 it was suggested that there exists a causal relationship between onset of cancer (oral cavity, pharynx, esophagus) and duration of the diet. However, it was shown that in celiac patients on a GFD for at least five years, this risk was not higher than that of the general population.

Clinical Manifestations of CD Predominantly Secondary to Malabsorption

Anemia

The association between anemia and CD is well known. However, even if it has been widely demonstrated that anemia could represent an isolated sign of CD, in patients with iron deficiency anemia refractory to iron therapy, the diagnosis of gluten intolerance is still infrequently recognized by both family physicians and hematologists.

Corazza et al. showed that 5% of patients who were referred to an outpatient hematology unit for isolated anemia had CD, and this prevalence rose to 8.5% when patients with macrocytic anemia or with microcytic anemia due to previous bleeding or responsive to oral iron therapy were excluded from the calculation [14]. Evidence of a strong association between anemia and CD has been shown even during childhood. In a study performed at the pediatric hospital of Pisa, Italy, 16 of 88 (18.18%) children who were consecutively evaluated for iron deficiency were EMA positive and underwent a subsequent biopsy confirming the underlying CD. Finally, it should be highlighted that iron deficiency anemia represents the most frequent sign suggestive of undiagnosed CD in screenings performed by the general practitioner. Other hematologic manifestations associated with CD include thrombocytosis linked to a functional hyposplenism and rarely erythroblastopenia likely of an immune-mediated nature. The prevalence of hyposplenism is increased in patients with CD especially if other autoimmune disorders are associated; therefore, these individuals are predisposed to an increased risk of sepsis with a high risk for pneumococcal sepsis [15].

Osteoporosis and Osteopenia

Osteoporosis and osteopenia are well-known complications detected in CD patients with an obscure pathogenesis. The prevalence of CD in adults with osteoporosis (3%) in one study was about 10 times higher than that of the general population (0.3%). Even more significant, however, are the many studies that show how in young and adult celiac patients on a free diet, bone mineral density is significantly lower than expected, while it tends to normalize with a GFD. Malabsorption, however, is not the only mechanism involved in the reduction of bone density: it has been shown that sera of celiac subjects, in a high percentage of cases (51.5%), test positive with immunofluorescence assays for the presence of antibodies directed against rat fetal bone structures, irrespective of the bone mineral density [16]. If these sera are then adsorbed with tissue transglutaminase, the pattern of fluorescence is greatly reduced until it disappears, indicating that the "anti-bone" antibodies are actually anti-tTG antibodies. It can then be concluded that bone loss in untreated celiac disease is likely the result of several factors: calcium malabsorption, lower milk intake due to possible lactose intolerance, secondary hyperparathyroidism, vitamin D malabsorption, or also the presence of autoantibodies directed against bone structures. It is particularly interesting to note that bone loss occurs in the same manner regardless of the presence of gastrointestinal symptoms, and that a GFD diet is consistently effective in correcting the bone density. It is well known that the bone density is inversely related to the risk of fractures and that untreated adult CD patients have a higher prevalence of fractures (21%) when compared to healthy peer controls (3%) [17]. It is possible that a GFD is less effective in restoring normal bone mineralization in elderly patients and this suggests the usefulness of CD screening in osteopenic subjects.

Immune-Mediated Clinical Manifestations of CD

Neurological Syndromes Associated with CD

Epilepsy

CD patients have a moderately higher risk (RR 1.43) than the general population to develop epilepsy. This risk was observed in 27 cases out of 100,000 and covers all ages including the pediatric age [18]. A rare form of epilepsy characterized by occipital calcifications seems to be the most typical type associated with CD. These are serpiginous calcifications of vascular origin. Before the CD-epilepsy-cerebral calcification (CE) syndrome was definitely recognized, some cases were classified as atypical Sturge-Weber syndrome given their similarity in cerebral calcifications with findings in real Sturge-Weber cases at computed tomography examination, but without facial angiomas or mental retardation. Clinically, patients present with patterns of partial occipital drug-resistant epilepsy, without clear signs of malabsorption. The relationship between the development of calcifications and CD has been unclear, while today there is evidence in favor of an autoimmune hypothesis based on the presence of autoantibodies directed against neurons and glial cells and high levels of anti-tTG6 in celiac patient sera [19]. In addition, there is strong evidence showing that a GFD can lead to better control of seizures and a reduction in the use of antiepileptic drugs and improved long-term prognosis, but only if it is started promptly and no later than elementary school age. CE may in fact evolve towards an epileptogenic encephalopathy. Initially, neuroimaging may be negative and calcifications appear secondarily. A lack of folate is however observed in almost all cases and it has been suggested to play a pathogenic role in the development of some intracranial calcifications which are indeed present, in other congenital and iatrogenic conditions characterized by low folacidemia.

Gluten Ataxia

In 1996, a group of British neurologists studied the surprisingly high prevalence (57%) of undiagnosed CD in patients with neurological disease of unknown origin. Most of these patients presented with ataxic disorders. In particular, approximately a quarter of patients with idiopathic ataxia showed serological evidence of sensitization to gluten. The same authors defined this condition as *gluten ataxia*, an idiopathic ataxia with evidence of sensitization to gluten. It is characterized by the insidious onset of predominantly gait ataxia, rarely associated with myoclonus and often associated with symptoms and signs suggestive of peripheral neuropathy usually affecting adult patients. Up to 60% of patients with gluten ataxia have evidence of cerebellar atrophy on magnetic resonance imaging.

By definition all gluten ataxia patients have positive IgG and/or IgA anti-gliadin antibodies, while anti-endomysium antibodies are present in only 22% of patients and anti-tTG antibodies are positive in up to 56% of patients. All patients have HLA DQ2 and DQ8 predisposition, while only a third presents with histological evidence of CD or with gastrointestinal symptoms [20]. The duration of exposure to gluten is apparently directly related to the severity of ataxia and indirectly related to the effectiveness of a GFD in reversing symptoms. In practice, this strongly underlines how in genetically predisposed individuals, gluten can induce an extraintestinal disease apart from overt enteropathy.

Experimental evidence suggests that there is an antibody cross-reactivity between antigenic epitopes on Purkinje cells and gluten peptides. Widespread deposits of IgA antibodies anti-tTG6 have been identified around the vessels of the cerebellum, pons and medulla of patients with gluten ataxia. The response to a GFD depends on the duration of ataxia as the progressive loss of Purkinje cells is irreversible. Diagnosis is not easy because only one third of patients have anti-IgA tTG2 and usually at titers less than those usually encountered in CD. Unlike celiac patients, patients with gluten ataxia show anti-tTG2 class IgG antibodies more frequently than anti-tTG2 class IgA.

Type 1 Diabetes Mellitus

Traditional studies, both in children and adults, have shown that CD occurs in patients with T1DM with a prevalence that varies from 4.4 to 11.1% compared with 0.5% of the general population [21]. The observation of an increased association between T1DM and CD supports the hypothesis that gluten might play a role in the pathogenesis of T1DM. The associated mechanism for these two diseases involves a shared genetic background (mainly linked to HLA) and an autoimmune pathogenic mechanism with the presence of organ-specific autoantibodies and infiltration of T lymphocytes to the site of the lesion. The classical severe presentation of CD rarely occurs in T1DM patients, and more often patients have few/mild symptoms of CD or are completely asymptomatic. In these T1DM patients usually CD diagnosis is achieved by means of routine blood screening. The effects of a GFD on the growth and T1DM metabolic control in the CD/T1DM patient are controversial. Adherence to a GFD by children with CD-T1DM has been reported generally below 50%, lower with respect to the 73% of CD patients without T1DM. Lower compliance is more frequent among asymptomatic adolescent CD/T1DM patients.

Dilated Cardiomyopathy

Dilated cardiomyopathy (DCM) is a complex disorder in which pathophysiologic and immunologic factors may play a role. An autoimmune pathogenetic mechanism is hypothesized and it involves the formation of autoantibodies directed against the α-myosin of cardiac muscle in addition to an association with a high expression of HLA class II on the endocardium and myocardium. This determines muscle damage, expansion of the ventricular chambers and/or an atrial defect and worsening of the heart's pumping ability. Previous small studies have suggested an increased prevalence of DCM in patients with CD and to confirm this finding a large population-based cohort study, was conducted on more than 29,000 CD patients. This nationwide study found a moderate, even if not statistically significant, increased risk of idiopathic DCM in patients with biopsy-verified CD [22].

Pathology of Reproduction: Fertility and Pregnancy

A possible causal relationship between untreated CD and reproductive problems (recurrent miscarriages, infertility) was first proposed in the 70s. Several studies have shown that women with CD on an unrestricted diet frequently have a shorter fertile period than the average, both because menarche is delayed and menopause is early. These women also have a lower than average number of children and a significantly higher number of abortions compared to women without CD. Ciacci et al. compared the reproductive life of 94 women with untreated CD with 31 celiac women on a GFD. In untreated women, the relative risk of abortion was 8.9 times higher and the risk of having low birth weight infants was increased 5.8 fold [23]. Also, in untreated celiac women the duration of breastfeeding (indirect index of mothers' health and nutrition) was 2.5 times shorter than in those who were on a GFD. Other studies have shown that women with CD who start a GFD exhibit a drastic reduction in the risk of abortions or complicated pregnancies.

Considering the high prevalence of "silent" CD as documented by screening of schoolchildren or blood donors, it is expected that about one in 100 pregnant women has CD. If we consider on one hand the risk of pregnancy morbidity in CD women and the high prevalence of CD in the general population even in comparison with rubella (0.01:1,000) and toxoplasmosis (0.5:1,000), it would seem reasonable to include an anti-tTG screening as "mandatory", at least during the first pregnancy [24]. Recently, however, the causal role of undiagnosed CD in determining an unfavorable evolution of pregnancy has been challenged [25].

Dermatitis Herpetiformis

Dermatitis herpetiformis (DH) is an autoimmune disease with a chronic-relapsing course, characterized by pruritic polymorphic lesions and typical histopathological, immunopathological, and serological findings. It is the main specific cutaneous manifestation of CD. Its prevalence ranges between 1:2,000 to 1:10,000 and even though it might affect patients of any age it is more frequent in adult patients.

The pathogenetic mechanism that triggers this cutaneous inflammatory response is linked to the presence of antibodies against an isoform of tTG present in the skin (tTG3) [26]. Skin lesions are predominantly associated with characteristic extensor surfaces, elbows, knees, and buttocks, which are the site of constant minor trauma. Only a minority of patients has gastrointestinal symptoms which are usually mild even if they are associated with villous atrophy in more than three-quarters of cases. The serological pattern is typical of CD. DH diagnosis is based on immunofluorescence demonstration on skin biopsy of fibrillar or granular deposits of IgA. Because of its well known association with CD, a diagnosis of DH assumes the presence of a gluten-sensitive enteropathy, and therefore an intestinal biopsy is not required. The skin lesions are gluten sensitive and disappear with a GFD.

Liver Disease Associated with CD

The liver is a glandular structure directly connected to the intestine via the portal system and therefore it directly receives through the portal blood nutrients and antigens that are absorbed and modified on the absorptive surface of the small intestine. Despite the possibility of an intuitive association between CD and hepatobiliary diseases, there is now sufficient evidence to support the fact that some hepatobiliary diseases are specifically associated with CD [27].

The association between CD and liver damage, was first reported in the late '70s. The variety of liver lesions may be schematically due to three conditions:

- Mild/moderate inflammatory damage, usually asymptomatic, although persistent, reversible with a GFD;
- More severe inflammatory damage, often symptomatic, evolving to fibrosis and cirrhosis, and generally insensitive to a GFD alone;
- Functional organ insufficiency favorably influenced with gluten withdrawal.

In addition, some hepatobiliary diseases of nonspecific inflammatory nature such as steatosis, nodular regenerative hyperplasia and hepatocellular carcinoma are sporadically associated with CD (table 3).

Table 3. CD associated liver disorders

Chronic nonspecific hepatitis (*celiac hepatitis*)
Autoimmune liver diseases:
• Autoimmune hepatitis type 1 and 2
• Primary biliary cirrhosis
• Autoimmune cholangitis
• Primary sclerosing cholangitis
• Overlap syndrome
Non alcoholic fatty liver disease
Acute liver disease
Cryptogenic cirrhosis
Nodular regenerative hyperplasia

Celiac Hepatitis

Elevation of transaminases is the most common laboratory abnormality seen at diagnosis in individuals genetically intolerant to gluten. In 1977 it was observed that 40% of adult patients with CD, had elevated transaminases at diagnosis and that this was generally reversible with gluten withdrawal. An assessment of liver histology showed in some cases chronic non-specific reactive hepatitis and in others a variable pathologic spectrum from steatosis to fibrosis to cirrhosis. This observation was subsequently confirmed in pediatric patients, where up to 60% of celiac patients with gastrointestinal symptoms, had a mild/moderate transaminase elevation at diagnosis generally sensitive to a GFD. These patients, when subjected to a liver biopsy showed preserved lobular architecture with a modest inflammatory infiltrate in the portal space and mild Kupffer cell hyperplasia [28].

An association between CD and chronic hepatobiliary disease was reported for the first time in 1986 in a teenager without gastrointestinal symptoms suggestive of CD, with cryptogenic and persistent transaminase elevation and histological features of mild/moderate inflammatory liver disease [29]. In this case, CD diagnosis was suggested by the finding of anti-reticulin autoantibodies. This observation was subsequently confirmed in asymptomatic children with cryptogenic elevated aminotransferase levels; in these patients a GFD determined transaminase normalization and improvement of histological features [30]. Furthermore, a gluten challenge was associated, once again, with an increase in aminotransferase levels. Subsequently, several retrospective studies in adults patients, confirmed these pediatric findings suggesting that about 9% of adult patients with persistent and cryptogenic hypertransaminasemia could have CD [31]. This condition of gluten-sensitive and gluten-dependent liver damage, defined as "celiac hepatitis" [32], is thus characterized by:

- the absence of clinical signs and/or symptoms suggestive of chronic liver disease;
- a moderate alteration of liver function tests limited to an increase in aminotransferase levels;
- histological features of moderate portal and lobular inflammation with Kupffer cell hyperplasia.

Once gluten has been withdrawn, normalization of liver enzymes is essential to confirm the celiac hepatitis diagnosis. Normalization of liver enzymes usually occurs within 6 months of starting a GFD, in some cases it may take place within 12 months. In case of lack of normalization of liver enzymes, an alternative diagnosis must be considered.

Celiac Disease and Autoimmune Liver Disease

Individuals with CD have a 2 to 6-fold greater risk to develop liver disease than the general population and the prevalence of CD in adults with chronic liver disease is about 15 times higher than that of the general population [33]. Celiac disease may, in particular, be associated with chronic liver diseases such as autoimmune diseases such as autoimmune ones: primary biliary cirrhosis (PBC), primary sclerosing cholangitis (PSC), autoimmune hepatitis (AIH) and all the overlapping conditions of these clinical entities [28]. The association between CD and PBC is widely described in adults, with a prevalence of CD among PBC patients ranging from 2.6 to 7%; also up to 3% of celiac patients may develop PBC. Gluten withdrawal does not alter, in any way, the evolution of biliary disease.

The relationship between CD and sclerosing cholangitis is supported by numerous observations with an epidemiological estimated risk in the celiac population, of about 4 times that of the general population. Regarding autoimmune hepatitis, the prevalence of CD in adults and children with AIH varies from 3.4 to 6.4%, with an 8-fold higher prevalence than the general population. In addition, of 909 children evaluated with CD, 1% was found to be affected by autoimmune hepatitis, in comparison with none in the control group [34]. A retrospective multicenter SIGENP study confirmed these data thus strengthening the belief that autoimmune liver disease is an extraintestinal "privileged" complication of CD [35]. This study found a CD prevalence greater than 16% in 140 pediatric patients with autoimmune liver diseases followed in Italian specialized centers for pediatric liver disease. Autoimmune hepatitis was the most prevalent condition, with a few rare cases of autoimmune cholangitis. In the majority of cases, the diagnosis of CD preceded that of autoimmune liver disease, although in almost all cases an increase of aminotransferases levels was already present, and was not modified with a GFD.

In a minority of cases, however, no evidence of hepatobiliary disease was found at diagnosis and autoimmune hepatitis presented as acute hepatitis, sometimes severe. In a third group of patients, the hepatobiliary disease was diagnosed before CD, as they were CD asymptomatic. Celiac disease diagnosis in these patients was accidental, usually secondary to a systematic serological screening of patients diagnosed with autoimmune liver disease.

Liver Diseases Associated with CD and Organ Failure

Cryptogenic liver disease with end-stage organ failure requiring a liver transplant has sporadically been reported in patients with CD. However, a 2002 study from Finland found an incidence of approximately 4 times the norm (4.3%) for individuals with undiagnosed CD, among patients who were candidates for liver transplantation: almost all of these patients had an autoimmune liver disease [36]. The surprising finding of this study was that in 3 out of 4 patients, a GFD had a favorable effect on hepatocellular function, possibly even preventing in progression to hepatic failure, even in cases in which liver transplantation was considered.

Pathogenesis of Liver Damage

The mechanisms for such a wide spectrum of liver damages in celiac patients are not defined, but it is possible that they can be integrated into a common pathogenetic pathway in which individual factors such as genetic predisposition, and environmental factors, such as early and long exposure to gluten, could influence the severity and reversibility of liver damage. It is well known that CD and some autoimmune liver disorders have a shared inherited predisposition for the expression of the same HLA class II molecules and haplotypes. In addition, the main CD genetic marker HLA-DQ2 is in strong linkage disequilibrium with HLA-DR3, which is the major HLA risk factor for autoimmune hepatitis [37]. Tissue transglutaminase plays a significant role in the process of fibrogenesis, apoptosis, and in general, inflammation. Tissue transglutaminase type 2 is the major autoantigen involved in the pathogenesis of CD and its ubiquitous distribution in different organs and tissues such as the skin, thyroid, pancreas, heart, bones, muscles, joints, reproductive system, peripheral and central nervous system and liver might explain some of the systemic manifestations of CD. In addition, individuals with CD have a significantly increased intestinal permeability which could facilitate the absorption of antigens from the intestinal lumen. These absorbed antigens interacting with self-antigens, such as TG2, could trigger the immune response to epitopes of common hepato-specific antigens in genetically predisposed individuals. This hypothesis is supported by the observation of extracellular deposits of anti-TG2 IgA in liver biopsies of patients with CD in the active phase [38].

The restoration of the intestinal mucosa permeability in celiac patients who are no longer exposed to gluten reduces the antigenic load, improving autoimmune liver disease control once remission has been induced by immunosuppressive therapy. This hypothesis seems to be supported by observations made in the recent study by SIGENP that relapses in patients with autoimmune liver disorders and CD seem closely related to the voluntary suspension of their GFD. Gluten withdrawal could have a favorable effect, helping patients with autoimmune hepatitis to maintain remission after immunosuppressive therapy discontinuation [39].

Diagnosis of Celiac Disease

Diagnosis of CD is based on serological testing by specific markers, and by histological analysis of duodenal biopsies. A diagnostic algorithm in the symptomatic and the asymptomatic patient based on new ESPGHAN guidelines is illustrated in figures 5 and 6.

HLA–DQ2 and HLA-DQ8 typing is a useful, but expensive tool to exclude CD in the case of a negative test result for both markers. Serologic screening is also recommended in all first-degree family members of patients who receive a diagnosis of CD.

Spectrum of Gluten Intolerance 29

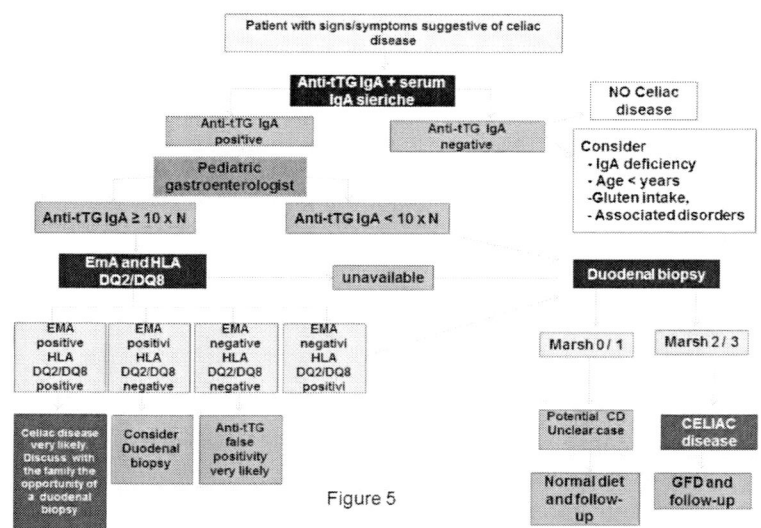

Figure 5. Diagnostic algorithm in the symptomatic patient with suspected CD.
GFD: gluten free diet; tTG: tissue transglutaminase; IgA: immunoglobulin A; HLA: human histocompatibility antigen.

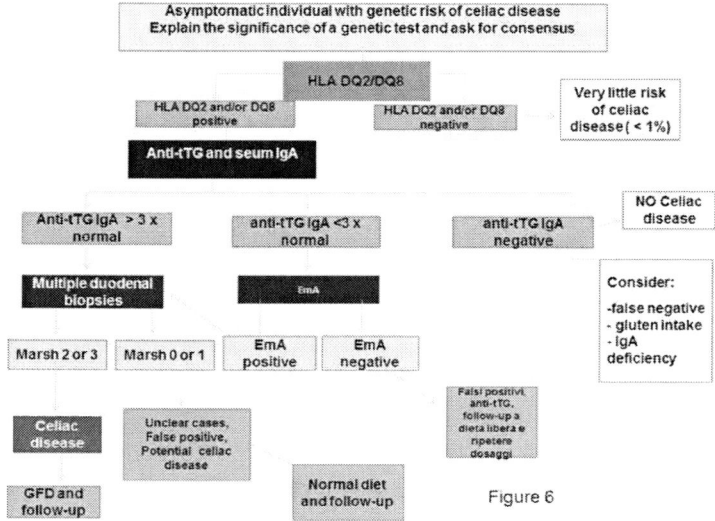

Figure 6. Diagnostic algorithm in the asymptomatic patient with possible CD.
GFD: gluten free diet; tTG: tissue transglutaminase; IgA: immunoglobulin A; HLA: human histocompatibility antigen.

Specific Antibody Tests

CD-specific antibody tests detect and measure the presence of immunoglobulin A (IgA) anti-tissue tranglutaminase-2 (anti-tTG2) antibody in the serum and the reactivity of anti-endomysial autoantibodies (EMA) (table 4). All diagnostic serologic testing should be performed in patients on a gluten containing diet.

- *Anti-tTG2* are circulating, gluten-dependent, autoantibodies that target transglutaminase 2, the principal self-antigen involved in the pathogenesis of CD. Tissue transglutaminase 2 is a calcium-dependent cytosolic enzyme belonging to the tissue transglutaminase family. In the extracellular space, TG2 is involved in the cell-extracellular matrix interactions and also in the remodeling and stabilization of the extracellular matrix. Tissue transglutaminase 2 is mainly expressed in the lamina propria, and its expression is up-regulated by various stimuli, such as mechanical stress or bacterial/viral infection. The enzyme catalyzes transamidation between a glutamine residue of a glutamine-donor protein and a lysine residue of a glutamine-acceptor protein, linking these proteins with a stable intermolecular isopeptide bond and increasing their rate of phagocytosis by antigen-presenting cells. Antibodies to tTG2 are present in the serum, but also in the jejunal juice and are produced solely in the intestinal mucosa. In CD, anti-tTG2 antibodies have been shown to influence the protein cross-linking enzymatic activity of TG2. It may also be hypothesized that binding of autoantibodies to TG2 also disturbs TG2 mediated cellular adhesion. It has also been shown that sub-epithelial blistering leading to loss of surface epithelial cells occurs in the celiac mucosa, coincident with findings indicating that the most pronounced IgA deposition is characteristically seen sub-epithelially. TG2 related IgA deposits in the morphologically normal jejunum have been shown to be predictive of forthcoming overt CD with villous atrophy. They may thus be regarded as a further marker of developing CD and CD latency, and a promising diagnostic tool in cases with low-grade enteropathy.

The search for IgA class anti-TG2 is the preferred single test for detection of CD in the primary care setting, because of its high sensitivity (97%) and specificity (91%) (table 4). This search should be performed in case of clinical suspicion of CD as well as in first-degree relatives of newly diagnosed CD patients. The test is most commonly based on an enzyme-linked immunosorbent assay. In comparison with anti-endomysial antibody, the anti-TG2 IgA assay has greater sensitivity and reproducibility.

IgA deficiency is more common in CD patients than in the general population. For subjects with low serum IgA levels (total serum IgA<0.2 µg/L), IgG class anti-TG2 should be evaluated. The anti-tTG2 titer correlates with the degree of mucosal damage.

- *Anti-endomysial antibodies (EMA)* are directed against the intermyofibril substance of smooth muscle, which may correspond either to a reticulin-like structure or a surface component of smooth muscle fibrils. These are detected by indirect immune fluorescence on monkey esophagus cells and on human umbilical cord cells as a substrate. The routine use of the EMA assay is limited by its high cost and technical expertise required. The EMA assay specificity is high (about 100%), but it is also IgA-based and the EMA IgG assay is not widely available. The EMA assay is mainly considered a confirmatory assay and should be used only in the case of borderline positive or possibly false positive results for anti-tissue transglutaminase antibodies, which are indicative of other autoimmune diseases, including T1DM.
- *Antibodies directed against native gliadin* are no longer recommended in serological testing for CD. However *antibodies directed against synthetic deamidated IgG class gliadin peptides* (anti-DPG), have a diagnostic role in IgA deficient patient with a suspicion of CD. Testing for anti-DPG (IgG may prove useful in EMA and anti-tTG negative patients and in IgA deficient patients when CD is suspected and in the screening of children younger than 2 years of age [6].

The use of rapid IgA anti-tTG assays based on serum or on whole blood drops has been recently proposed. These tests have shown high sensitivity and specificity ranging from 90.2 to 100% and 94.9 to 100%, respectively. These assays offer the general practitioner who suspects a possible case of CD, the possibility of looking for anti-tTG antibodies in his own medical office during a standard visit and the possibility of evaluating dietary compliance in an ambulatory setting at a satisfyingly low cost [40].

Table 4. Celiac disease screening: serological testing

Test	Mean sensitivity	Mean Specificity	Use
Anti-tTG IgA	94 %	97%	Testing
Anti-tTG IgG	Variable (12-99%)	Variable (86-99%)	IgA deficiency
Anti-EMA IgA	>90%	98%	Confirmatory test
Anti-DPG IgG	>90 %	>90%	IgA deficiency and children <2 years
HLA-DQ2 and HLA DQ8	91%	54%	High negative predictive value

Small Bowel Biopsy

An upper endoscopy with small bowel biopsy is a critical component of the diagnostic evaluation for individuals with suspected CD and is recommended in most patients to confirm the diagnosis [41]. The availability of CD-specific serological tests and their increasing role in diagnostics has questioned the need for a small bowel biopsy in some particular settings such as in young patients. A recent guideline promulgated by the European Society for Pediatric Gastroenterology, Hepatology and Nutrition (ESPGHAN) proposed to avoid any intestinal biopsy in children who meet the following criteria: characteristic signs and symptoms of CD, anti-tTG IgA levels higher than 10 times the upper normal limit confirmed by a positive EMA assay, and the presence of HLA-DQ2/DQ8.

The efficacy of this strategy has been retrospectively evaluated in 150 symptomatic children with suspected CD, with a positive predictive value, of the so-called triple test, (immunoglobulin A-tissue transglutaminase antibody, anti-endomysial antibody, and HLA genotype) of 97.4% for patients with Marsh 2 or 3 histological lesions. The other three cases

(2.6%) who had Marsh 0 or 1 lesions on small bowel biopsy were considered false-positives for the triple test. However, at follow-up, all three children developed histological damage after a gluten challenge leading to a final 100% positive predictive value of the triple test [42]. Recent guidelines issued from other International societies, however, still consider the demonstration of histological changes associated with the disease mandatory to confirm the diagnosis [41]. Prospective studies to validate ESPGHAN recommendations are ongoing.

All duodenal biopsies are performed nowadays by endoscopic examination. Biopsies performed with the Crosby-Watson capsule by perioral route are considered outdated and are no longer performed.

Assessment of the biopsy requires proper orientation of the specimen. Elementary lesions associated with CD include:

- *Intraepithelial lymphocytosis*: a number of intraepithelial T lymphocytes (IEL) greater than 30 per 100 enterocytes;
- *Crypt hyperplasia:* extension of the regenerative epithelial crypts associated with changes in the presence of more than 1 mitosis per crypt;
- *Villous atrophy:* decrease in villous height, alteration of normal crypt/villous ratio (3:1) until total disappearance of villi.

None of these elementary CD lesions is exclusive; moreover lesions may be patchy, for this reason, multiple biopsies of the duodenum (at least one biopsy of the bulb and four of the distal duodenum) are recommended to confirm the diagnosis [41]. In children, adding biopsies of the bulb increase the diagnostic power because about 10% of them have villous atrophy exclusively located in the duodenal bulb [43].

Histological changes in CD can be classified according to Marsh or Marsh modified staging (Oberhuber) [44].

Marsh classification identifies three distinct entities:

Type 1 or infiltrative lesion: characterized by normal villous and crypt architecture, normal villous/crypt ratio (3:1) and by an increased number of intraepithelial lymphocytes (greater than 30 per 100 epithelial cells);

Type 2 or hyperplastic lesion: characterized by normal villous architecture (like type 1), hyperplasia of the glandular element with an increased number of mitoses and increased intraepithelial lymphocytes (like type 1);

Type 3 or destructive lesion: characterized by varying degrees of villous atrophy associated with hyperplasia of the glandular crypt and increased intraepithelial lymphocytes (like type 1 and 2 lesions). An amendment to this classification was proposed by Oberhuber et al. [44] who divided the Marsh type 3 lesion into three subgroups according to the severity of villous atrophy: ***3a*** mild villous atrophy and pathological increase of IELs; ***3b*** moderate villous atrophy and pathological increase of IELs; ***3c*** total villous atrophy and pathological increase of IELs (figure 7).

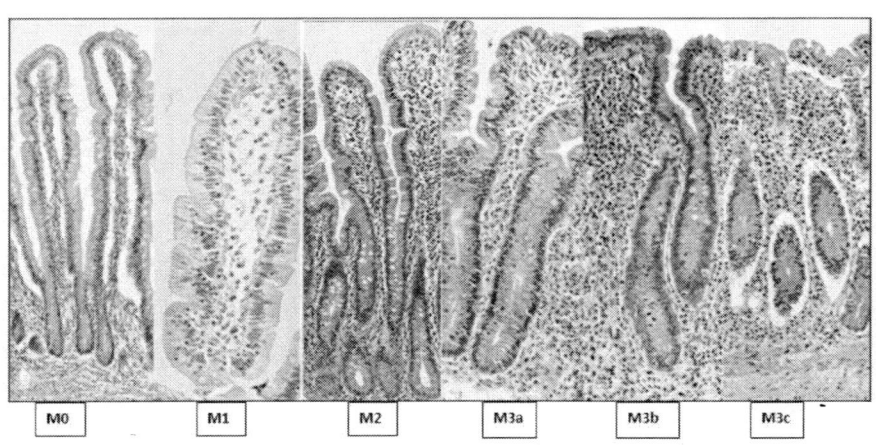

Figure 7. Marsh modified (Oberhuber) classification [44]. M0= normal villus; M1= increase of IELs; M2 increase of intraepithelial lymphocytes and glandular crypt hyperplasia; M3a partial villous atrophy; M3b subtotal villous atrophy; M3c total villous atrophy.

In an attempt to simplify the communication between pathologists and clinicians, a new histological classification has recently been proposed by Corazza and Villanacci [45, 46] where the lesions that characterize CD have been divided into two categories: *non-atrophic (grade A)* and *atrophic (grade B)*. *Grade A* lesions are characterized by a pathological increase in intraepithelial lymphocytes, best recognized by the use of immunohistochemical techniques. *Atrophic Grade B* lesions are further subdivided into: *Grade B1*, in which the villus/crypt ratio is less than 3:1 and villi are still identifiable, and *Grade B2* in which the villi are no longer identifiable.

When evaluating the duodenal mucosa the pathologist should:

1. Carefully assess the orientation of the biopsies, to correctly identify all intestinal layers and to avoid false positive results (e.g., normal mucosa with an atrophic appearance in a specimen that has not been cut longitudinally);
2. Consider whether the villus/crypt ratio of at least 3:1 is respected;
3. Carefully count the number of lymphocytes on the surface coating the epithelium and carry out additional immunohistochemical evaluation with CD3;
4. Classify the lesion following a validated classification.

If frozen material is available, immunohistochemical typing for the gamma-delta receptor of T lymphocytes should be carried out. In normal conditions this receptor is not expressed by more than 2-3% of T lymphocytes while in CD it may reach 20–30%.

The detection of sub epithelial anti-tissue transglutaminase antibody IgA deposits by means of double immunofluorescence may be useful in patients with an uncertain diagnosis, such as patients with negative serological results and positive results on biopsy [47].

Marsh type 1 lesion interpretation is crucial in distinguishing early gluten-related damage from other causes. Borderline lymphocytic infiltration (between 25 and 29 intraepithelial lymphocytes per 100 enterocytes) is common in the general population and most patients with lymphocytic duodenosis (≥30 intraepithelial lymphocytes per 100 enterocytes) and does not belong to the spectrum of CD.

Table 5 shows that in addition to CD, there are a number of pathological conditions that have the same morphological aspects as CD in its early stages. These conditions include hypersensitivity to other foods (milk, soybeans, etc.), infections (*Helicobacter pylori*, *Giardia*, etc.), immunodeficiencies and autoimmune diseases (Hashimoto thyroiditis, systemic lupus erythematosus, rheumatoid arthritis, etc.), and chronic idiopathic inflammatory bowel colitis or colitis with a different etiology, such as lymphocytic and collagenous colitis.

Table 5. Causes of proximal small intestinal intraepithelial lymphocytosis with normal villus architecture

Non-gluten food hypersensitivity (e.g., cow's milk, soy products)
Infections (e.g., viral enteritis, *Giardia*, *Cryptosporidium*, *Helicobacter pylori*)
Bacterial overgrowth
Immune deficiency (e.g., IgA deficiency, common variable immunodeficiency)
Autoimmune disorders (e.g., Hashimoto thyroiditis, rheumatoid arthritis, SLE, autoimmune enteropaty)
Chronic inflammatory bowel disease
Lymphocytic and collagenous colitis

Unlike what occurs in children, there is considerable evidence that CD in adults, especially if diagnosed late and even more, so if not dealt with by a timely and rigorous GFD, is burdened by potentially severe complications such as:

- *Collagenous sprue:* The patient does not respond to a GFD and histology shows fibrous tissue in the intestinal wall at the level of the superficial sub-epithelial layer. This morphological pattern is very similar to the collagenous colitis condition described in the colon;
- *Refractory sprue:* This condition reproduces the same clinical picture as collagenous sprue, but can be identified by immunohistochemical staining, demonstrating that T lymphocytes, which under normal conditions express CD3 and CD8, in this case express only CD3 and not CD8;
- *Ulcerative jejunoileitis:* Presence of extensive ulceration of the intestinal mucosa, often related to refractory sprue;
- *Lymphoma:* This complication should always be suspected when histology shows the prevalence of atypical monomorphous lymphocytic elements. In this case it is useful to carry out immunophenotyping of the lymphoid population, which is almost always type T.

Finally, in case of non-CD villous atrophy, other diagnostic options should be included in the differential diagnosis (table 6).

Table 6. Other causes of villous atrophy in the duodenum

Malnutrition
Small bowel bacterial overgrowth
Parasitic infection (eg. giardiasis, criptosporidiosis, microsporidiosis)
Viral infections (eg. cytomegalovirus, herpes virus)
Tropical sprue
Hypogammaglobinemic sprue
Autoimmune enteropathy
Whipple disease
Intestinal tuberculosis
Collagenous sprue
Eosinophilic enteritis
Crohn's disease
Cow's milk /soy protein intolerance
Radiation enteritis
Intestinal lymphoma
Graft versus host disease
Acquired immune deficiency syndrome enteropathy

Genetic Testing

Celiac disease is closely associated with the presence of HLA-DQ heterodimers DQ2 (encoded by alleles A1*05 and B1*02) and DQ8 (encoded by alleles A1*03 and B1*0302). HLA DQ2 ($\approx$ 95%) or HLA DQ8 ($\approx$5%) are present in almost all patients with CD. This test has a high negative predictive value (>99%) which means that the disease is very unlikely to develop in subjects who are negative for both HLA-DQ2 and HLA-DQ8. Among very few patients not carrying these heterodimers, the majority encoded half of the HLA-DQ2 heterodimer.

HLA DQ2/8 testing should not be used in the initial CD diagnosis due to its high cost and the low positive predictive value ($\approx$ 12%), but should be used to rule out CD in selected clinical presentations such as:

- Equivocal histological findings (Marsh 1-2) in seronegative patients;
- Evaluation of patients on a GFD not tested for CD before starting the diet;
- Evaluation of at-risk persons to exclude a genetic predisposition to CD such as in children with Down's syndrome. A negative result for both HLA-DQ2 and DQ8 would reassure most parents about the absence of a genetic risk for CD development.

The utility of HLA testing in other at-risk groups such as patients with T1DM or first-degree family members of patients diagnosed with CD is uncertain due to the high proportion of subjects carrying the CD susceptibility alleles. In fact, HLA DQ2/8 is present in approximately 30-35% of the general population and in 60-70% of 1st degree relatives of patients with CD, but approximately only 10% of them will develop CD.

Treatment and Follow-Up

A strict GFD is the only effective treatment for CD and will result in resolution of symptoms (when present), disappearance of "celiac" autoantibodies in the serum, and repair of intestinal mucosal damage usually within 24 months. Moreover, a GFD improves the CD patient's nutritional parameters such as body mass index and bone mineral density.

Individuals diagnosed with CD should adhere to a GFD for life, avoiding all products containing wheat, barley and rye. Pure oats, uncontaminated by other grains containing gluten, appear to be safely tolerated by the majority of people with CD. However, when oats are introduced to the diet in an individual with CD a careful follow up is mandatory to monitor for signs of clinical and serological relapse.

Life-long compliance to a GFD is however difficult and expensive. Moreover, complete elimination of gluten from the diet is not possible due to contamination with trace amounts of gluten. The *International Codex Alimentarius* defines "gluten-free" foods as having less than 20 parts per million (ppm) gluten (about 10 ppm gliadin). The lowest quantity of gluten known to be responsible for mucosal damage ranges from 10 to 50 mg per day. This suggests that an amount of gluten less than 10 mg per day is unlikely to cause damage in most patients. Even with these numerical considerations though, some patients with CD may be hyper-sensitive, and react after only a single ingestion of minute amounts of gluten.

Failure to adhere to a GFD carries a risk for adverse health consequences and increased mortality. Mortality is mainly related to an increased risk of malignancy. B-cell and T-cell non-Hodgkin lymphomas and in particular T-cell lymphomas are the most common malignancy diagnosed in CD patients. Strict avoidance of gluten is difficult, in particular, in Mediterranean countries where gluten consumption in the normal diet is high. Compliance to a GFD may be problematic in adolescence and in asymptomatic children diagnosed by systematic screening. For these reasons, individuals with CD should be monitored annually for adherence to the GFD by a health care practitioner with knowledge of CD. Verification of the disappearance of CD-specific autoantibodies is crucial during follow up; a persistent positive serology (anti-tTG2 and anti-DPG antibody) one year after starting a GFD suggests gluten contamination. Monitoring for adherence should be based on a diet survey as serology is not accurate enough to detect minor gluten contamination.

Finally, recent advances in the "non-dietary" treatment of CD include engineering gluten-free grains, degrading immunodominant gliadin peptides, decreasing intestinal permeability and inducing oral tolerance to gluten with a therapeutic vaccine.

- Plant breeding programs and/or transgenic technologies may lead to the production of wheat that is devoid of biologically active peptide sequences. The identification of specific epitopes may also provide a target for immunomodulation of antigenic peptides.
- Because of their high-proline content, gliadin peptides are highly resistant to digestion by pancreatic and brush border proteases. Supplementary enzyme therapy with bacterial endopeptidases has been proposed to promote complete digestion of cereal proteins and thus destroy T-cell multipotent epitopes. One of these enzyme formulations is currently in clinical trials and has shown promising safety and efficacy data. It remains to be assessed whether the residual amount of undigested gluten can cause harm in the long term. An alternative approach to reduce gluten toxicity is based on

- a pretreatment of whole gluten or gluten-containing food with bacterial-derived peptidase. Enzymatic detoxification of gluten has the potential to be an effective method for producing more palatable gluten-free products.
- Together with the gut-associated lymphoid tissue and the neuroendocrine network, the intestinal epithelial barrier, with its intercellular tight junctions, controls the equilibrium between tolerance and immunity to non-self antigens. When the trafficking of macromolecules is dysregulated, in genetically susceptible individuals, both intestinal and extra intestinal autoimmune disorders can occur. Small intestinal permeability abnormalities are seen in untreated CD patients, which return to normal on a GFD. A zonulin inhibitor (larazotide acetate) has been tested in a double blind, randomized placebo-controlled human clinical trial to determine its safety, tolerability, and preliminary efficacy. Larazotide was shown to be well tolerated and appears to reduce gluten-induced intestinal barrier dysfunction, proinflammatory cytokine production, and gastrointestinal symptoms in celiac patients.
- Selective inhibition of tTG in the small intestine might represent a therapeutically useful strategy for countering the immunotoxic response to dietary gluten in CD. The substitution of a glutamine residue with 6-diazo-5-oxo-norleucine transforms an immunodominant gluten peptide into a potent inhibitor of tissue transglutaminase. However, the efficacy and side effects of tTG inhibitors are unknown.

All these investigational therapies are in the research stage and are generally being considered as "adjunct" therapies to a GFD and not as substitutes at this point in time. It should be emphasized that treated CD is a benign condition and dietary treatment is safe, although strenuous. Therefore, any new approach must first demonstrate a safety profile equivalent to that of the GFD but with the advantage of increased compliance.

WHEAT ALLERGY

Wheat allergy (WA) is defined as an adverse IgE mediated reaction occurring minutes to hours after gluten ingestion. WA is a classic food allergy affecting the skin, and gastrointestinal or respiratory tract. More rare clinical manifestations of WA include wheat-dependent, exercise-induced anaphylaxis induced by a specific type of wheat protein, the ω_5-gliadins, occupational asthma (baker's asthma) associated with rhinitis and contact urticaria. The prevalence of sensitization to wheat in a North-European pediatric population varies between 0.5 and 4%. Wheat respiratory allergy and rhinitis is one of the most common and well-characterized forms of occupational asthma, and is induced by inhalation of wheat and cereal flour (4% of bakery apprentices). Diagnosis is based on skin prick tests and the demonstration of specific IgE antibodies.

FPIES (*Food Protein Enterocolitis Syndrome*) is a non-IgE-mediated gastrointestinal food hypersensitivity thought to be cell-mediated, although the exact pathophysiologic mechanism is unknown. FPIES typically presents in infants with debilitating vomiting, diarrhea, dehydration, pallor and lethargy and in 10-20% of cases, it presents with severe hypotension occurring 1 to 6 hours after ingesting the offending food. The most common offending foods are cow's milk, soy, rice and more rarely wheat. Diagnosis is based primarily on clinical history and, when unclear, physician-supervised oral food challenges. FPIES is usually outgrown by school age. Although management remains avoidance of the offending food, observations that FPIES natural history varies for different foods have redefined the timing of reintroduction. Early recognition of FPIES and removal of the offending food are imperative to prevent misdiagnosis and mismanagement of symptoms that may mimic other causes.

NON CELIAC (NON- WHEAT) GLUTEN SENSITIVITY

The increasing number of patients worldwide who are sensitive to dietary wheat (gluten), without evidence of CD or wheat allergy has contributed to the identification of a new gluten-related syndrome defined as non-celiac gluten sensitivity [48]. Non celiac gluten sensitivity (NCGS), originally described in the 1980s and recently "re-discovered", is a disorder characterized by intestinal (diarrhea, abdominal pain) and extra-intestinal symptoms related to the ingestion of gluten (wheat)-containing food, in subjects that are not affected with either CD or wheat allergy. Gastrointestinal and extra intestinal symptoms occur shortly after the ingestion of gluten and improve or disappear when gluten is withdrawn from the diet. These symptoms recur when gluten is reintroduced. Many aspects of this syndrome remain unknown; in particular its prevalence in the general population is highly variable, ranging from 0.63% to 6%. Lack of biomarkers is still a major limitation of clinical studies, making it difficult to differentiate NCGS from other gluten related disorders. This entity was also recently reported in children [49].

Also because diagnostic biomarkers have not yet been identified, a double-blind placebo-controlled gluten challenge is currently the diagnostic method with the highest accuracy.

Recent evidence showed that when patients with NCGS and irritable bowel syndrome were assigned to a diet with reduced content of fermentable, poorly absorbed, short-chain carbohydrates (fermentable, oligo-, di-, monosaccharides, and polyols [FODMAPs]), gastrointestinal symptoms consistently and significantly improved. Furthermore, they significantly worsened when their diets included gluten or whey protein, although there was not an evidence for a dose-dependent effects of gluten [50].

CONCLUSION

Gluten is one of the most abundant and diffusely spread dietary components. Gluten may provoke a wide range of adverse reactions, and CD is the most well characterized gluten-related disorder.

Patients with symptoms and signs suggestive of malabsorption, patients with an unexplained elevation of serum aminotransferase activity, patients with type I diabetes with digestive symptoms and first degree-family members of an individual with a confirmed diagnosis of CD, should be tested for CD while on a gluten containing diet, and IgA anti-tTG antibodies with associated serum total IgA should be measured to avoid confounding IgA deficiency results.

The confirmation of CD diagnosis should be based on a combination of findings including medical history, physical examination, serology and histological analysis of multiple duodenal biopsies. In children, in selected cases, the intestinal biopsy may be avoided.

If the suspicion of CD is high, an intestinal biopsy should be performed even if serology is negative.

HLA DQ2/8 should be included in diagnostic work up for CD only in selected cases and should not be used routinely.

Individuals with CD should strictly avoid all products containing protein from wheat, barley and rye. Pure oats appear to be safely tolerated, but an accurate follow-up is necessary in case of frequent oat consumption.

Children with CD should be monitored regularly for normal growth and development, appearance of symptoms, and adherence to GFD. Monitoring adherence to GFD should be based on a combination of personal and dietetic history and serology.

A diagnosis of non-celiac gluten sensitivity should be considered only when CD has been excluded by appropriate testing.

REFERENCES

[1] Fasano A; Catassi C. Celiac disease. *N Engl J Med* 2012; 367: 2419-2426.

[2] Van Berge-Henegouwen GP; Mulder CJ. Pioneer in the gluten free diet: Willem-Karel Dicke 1905-1962, over 50 years of gluten free diet. *Gut* 1993; 34: 1473-1475.

[3] Meeuwisse GW. Round table discussion. Diagnostic criteria in coeliac disease. *Acta Paediatr* 1970; 59: 461-463.

[4] McNeish AS; Harms HK; Rey J; Shmerling DH; Visakorpi JK; Walker-Smith JA. The diagnosis of celiac disease. A commentary on the current practices of members of the European Society for Paediatric Gastroenterology and Nutrition (ESPGAN). *Arch Dis Child* 1979; 54: 783-786.

[5] Report of Working Group of European Society of Paediatric Gastroenterology and Nutrition. Revised criteria for diagnosis of coeliac disease. *Arch Dis Child* 1990; 65: 909-911.

[6] Husby S; Koletzko S; Korponay-Szabó IR; Mearin ML; Phillips A; Shamir R; Troncone R; Giersiepen K; Branski D; Catassi C; Lelgeman M; Mäki M; Ribes-Koninckx C; Ventura A; Zimmer KP; ESPGHAN Working Group on Coeliac Disease Diagnosis; ESPGHAN Gastroenterology Committee; European Society for Pediatric Gastroenterology, Hepatology, and Nutrition. European Society for Pediatric Gastroenterology, Hepatology, and Nutrition guidelines for the diagnosis of coeliac disease. *J Pediatr Gastroenterol Nutr* 2012; 54: 136-160.

[7] Bai JC; Fried M; Corazza GR; Schuppan D; Farthing M; Catassi C; Greco L; Cohen H; Ciacci C; Eliakim R; Fasano A; González A; Krabshuis JH; LeMair A; World Gastroenterology Organization. World Gastroenterology Organisation Global Guidelines on Celiac Disease. *J Clin Gastroenterol* 2013; 47: 121-125.

[8] Ludvigsson JF; Leffler DA; Bai JC. The Oslo definitions for coeliac disease and related terms. *Gut* 2013; 62: 43–52.

[9] Reilly NR; Green PH. Epidemiology and clinical presentations of celiac disease. *Semin Immunopathol* 2012 ; 34: 473-478.

[10] Bourgey M; Calcagno G; Tinto N; Gennarelli D; Margaritte-Jeannin P; Greco L; Limongelli MG; Esposito O; Marano C; Troncone R; Spampanato A; Clerget-Darpoux F; Sacchetti L. HLA related genetic risk for coeliac disease. *Gut* 2007; 56: 1054-1059.

[11] Green PH; Cellier C. Celiac disease. *N Engl J Med* 2007; 357: 1731-1743.

[12] Tosco A; Salvati VM; Auricchio R; Maglio M; Borrelli M; Coruzzo A; Paparo F; Boffardi M; Esposito A; D'Adamo G; Malamisura B; Greco L; Troncone R. Natural history of potential celiac disease in children. *Clin Gastroenterol Hepatol* 2011; 9: 320-325.

[13] Not T; Ziberna F; Vatta S; Quaglia S; Martelossi S; Villanacci V; Marzari R; Florian F; Vecchiet M; Sulic AM; Ferrara F; Bradbury A; Sblattero D; Ventura A. Cryptic genetic gluten intolerance revealed by intestinal antitransglutaminase antibodies and response to gluten-free diet. *Gut* 2011 ;60: 1487-1493.

[14] Corazza GR; Valentini RA; Andreani ML; D'Anchino M; Leva MT; Ginaldi L; De Feudis L; Quaglino D; Gasbarrini G. Subclinical coeliac disease is a frequent cause of iron-deficiency anaemia. *Scand J Gastroenterol* 1995; 30: 153-156.

[15] Ludvigsson JF; Olén O; Bell M; Ekbom A; Montgomery SM. Coeliac disease and risk of sepsis. *Gut* 2008; 57: 1074-1080.
[16] Sugai E; Cherñavsky A; Pedreira S; Smecuol E; Vazquez H; Niveloni S; Mazure R; Mauriro E; Rabinovich GA; Bai JC. Bone-specific antibodies in sera from patients with celiac disease: characterization and implications in osteoporosis. *J Clin Immunol* 2002; 22: 353-362.
[17] Sánchez MI; Mohaidle A; Baistrocchi A; Matoso D; Vázquez H; González A; Mazure R; Maffei E; Ferrari G; Smecuol E; Crivelli A; de Paula JA; Gómez JC; Pedreira S; Mauriño E; Bai JC. Risk of fracture in celiac disease: gender, dietary compliance, or both? *World J Gastroenterol* 2011; 17: 3035-3042.
[18] Ludvigsson JF; Zingone F; Tomson T; Ekbom A; Ciacci C. Increased risk of epilepsy in biopsy-verified celiac disease: a population-based cohort study. *Neurology* 2012; 78: 1401-1407.
[19] Johnson AM; Dale RC; Wienholt L; Hadjivassiliou M; Aeschlimann D; Lawson JA. Coeliac disease, epilepsy, and cerebral calcifications: association with TG6 autoantibodies. *Dev Med Child Neurol* 2013; 55: 90-93.
[20] Hadjivassiliou M; Sanders DS; Woodroofe N; Williamson C; Grünewald RA. Gluten ataxia. *Cerebellum* 2008; 7: 494-498.
[21] Camarca ME; Mozzillo E; Nugnes R; Zito E; Falco M; Fattorusso V; Mobilia S; Buono P; Valerio G; Troncone R; Franzese A. Celiac disease in type 1 diabetes mellitus. *Ital J Pediatr* 2012; 38: 10.
[22] Emilsson L; Andersson B; Elfström P; Green PH; Ludvigsson JF. Risk of idiopathic dilated cardiomyopathy in 29000 patients with celiac disease. *J Am Heart Assoc* 2012; 1: e001594.
[23] Ciacci C; Cirillo M; Auriemma G; Di Dato G; Sabbatini F; Mazzacca G. Celiac disease and pregnancy outcome. *Am J Gastroenterol* 1996; 91: 718-722.
[24] Martinelli P; Troncone R; Paparo F; Torre P; Trapanese E; Fasano C; Lamberti A; Budillon G; Nardone G; Greco L. Coeliac disease and unfavourable outcome of pregnancy. *Gut* 2000; 46: 332-335.
[25] Greco L; Veneziano A; Di Donato L; Zampella C; Pecoraro M; Paladini D; Paparo F; Vollaro A; Martinelli P. Undiagnosed coeliac disease does not appear to be associated with unfavourable outcome of pregnancy. *Gut* 2004; 53: 149-151.

[26] Bonciani D; Verdelli A; Bonciolini V; D'Errico A; Antiga E; Fabbri P; Caproni M. Dermatitis herpetiformis: from the genetics to the development of skin lesions. *Clin Dev Immunol* 2012; 2012: 239691.
[27] Duggan JM; Duggan AE. Systematic review: the liver in celiac disease. *Aliment Pharmacol Ther* 2005; 21: 515-518.
[28] Rubio-Tapia A; Murray JA. The liver in celiac disease. *Hepatology* 2007; 46: 1650-1658.
[29] Maggiore G; De Giacomo C; Scotta MS; Sessa F. Celiac disease presenting as chronic hepatitis in a girl. *J Pediatr Gastroenterol Nutr* 1986; 5: 501-503.
[30] Vajro P; Fontanella A; Mayer M; De Vincenzo A; Terracciano LM; D'Armiento M; Vecchione R. Elevated serum aminotransferase activity as an early manifestation of gluten sensitive enteropathy. *J Pediatr* 1993; 122: 416-419.
[31] Volta U; De Franceschi L; Lari F; Molinaro N; Zoli M; Bianchi FB. Coeliac disease hidden by cryptogenic hypertransaminasemia. *Lancet* 1998; 352: 26-29.
[32] Maggiore G; Caprai S. The liver in celiac disease. *J Pediatr Gastroenterol Nutr* 2003; 37: 117-119.
[33] Ludvigson JF; Elfström P; Broomé U; Ekbom A; Montgomery SM. Celiac disease and risk of liver disease: a general population-based study. *Clin Gastroenterol Hepatol* 2007; 5: 63-69.
[34] Ventura A; Magazzu G; Greco L. Duration of exposure to gluten and risk for autoimmune disorders in patients with celiac disease. *Gastroenterology* 1999; 117: 297-303.
[35] Caprai S; Vajro P; Ventura A; Maggiore G and the SIGENP study group for autoimmune disorders in celiac disease. Autoimmune liver disease associated with celiac disease in childhood: a multicenter study. *Clin Gastroenterol Hepatol* 2008; 6: 803-806.
[36] Kaukinen K, Halme L, Collin P; Färkkilä M; Mäki M; Vehmanen P; Partanen J; Höckerstedt K. Coeliac disease in patients with severe liver disease: gluten free diet may reverse hepatic failure. *Gastroenterology* 2002; 122: 881-888.
[37] Volta A. Pathogenesis and clinical significance of liver injury in celiac disease. *Clin Rev Allergy Immunol* 2009; 36: 62-70.
[38] Korponay-Szabo IR; Halttunen T; Szalai Z; Laurila K; Király R; Kovács JB; Fésüs L; Mäki M. In vivo targeting of intestinal and

extraintestinal transglutaminase 2 by coeliac autoantibodies. *Gut* 2004; 53: 641-648.

[39] Nastasio S; Sciveres M; Riva S; Filippeschi IP; Vajro P; Maggiore G. Celiac disease associated-autoimmune hepatitis in childhood: long term response to treatment. *J Pediatr Gastroenterol Nutr* 2013; 56: 671-674.

[40] Nemec G; Ventura A; Stefano M; Di Leo G; Baldas V; Tommasini A; Ferrara F; Taddio A; Città A; Sblattero D; Marzari R; Not T. Looking for celiac disease: diagnostic accuracy of two rapid commercial assays. *Am J Gastroenterol* 2006; 101: 1597-1600.

[41] Rubio-Tapia A; Hill ID; Kelly CP; Calderwood AH; Murray JA. ACG Clinical Guidelines: diagnosis and management of celiac disease. *Am J Gastroenterol* 2013; 108: 656-676.

[42] Klapp G; Masip E; Bolonio M; Donat E; Polo B; Ramos D; Ribes-Koninckx C. Celiac disease: the new proposed ESPGHAN diagnostic criteria do work well in a selected population. *J Pediatr Gastroenterol Nutr* 2013; 56: 251-256.

[43] Bonamico M; Thanasi E; Mariani P; Nenna R; Luparia RP; Barbera C; Morra I; Lerro P; Guariso G; De Giacomo C; Scotta S; Pontone S; Carpino F; Magliocca FM; Società Italiana di Gastroenterologica, Epatologia, e Nutrizione Pediatrica. for the Società Italiana di Gastroenterologia, Epatologia, e Nutrizione Pediatrica. Duodenal bulb biopsies in celiac disease: a multicenter study. *J Pediatr Gastroenterol Nutr* 2008; 47: 618-622.

[44] Oberhuber G; Granditsch G; Vogelsang H. The histopathology of coeliac disease: time for a standardized report scheme for pathologists. *Eur J Gastroenterol Hepatol* 1999; 11: 1185-1194.

[45] Villanacci V; Ceppa P; Tavani E; Vindigni C; Volta U; Gruppo Italiano Patologi Apparato Digerente (GIPAD); Società Italiana di Anatomia Patologica e Citopatologia Diagnostica/International Academy of Pathology, Italian division (SIAPEC/IAP). Coeliac disease: the histology report. *Dig Liver Dis* 2011; 43 Suppl 4: S385-S395.

[46] Corazza GR; Villanacci V. Coeliac disease. *J Clin Pathol* 2005; 58: 573-574.

[47] Salmi TT; Collin P; Korponay-Szabó IR; Laurila K; Partanen J; Huhtala H; Király R; Lorand L; Reunala T; Mäki M; Kaukinen K.

Endomysial antibody-negative coeliac disease: clinical characteristics and intestinal autoantibody deposits. *Gut* 2006; 55:1746-1753.

[48] Catassi C; Bai JC; Bonaz B; Bouma G; Calabrò A; Carroccio A; Castillejo G; Ciacci C; Cristofori F; Dolinsek J; Francavilla R; Elli L; Green P; Holtmeier W; Koehler P; Koletzko S; Meinhold C; Sanders D; Schumann M; Schuppan D; Ullrich R; Vécsei A; Volta U; Zevallos V; Sapone A; Fasano A. Non-celiac gluten sensitivity: the new frontier of gluten related disorders. *Nutrients* 2013 ; 5 :3839-3853.

[49] Francavilla R; Cristofori F; Castellaneta S; Polloni C; Albano V; Dellatte S; Indrio F; Cavallo L; Catassi C. Clinical, serologic, and histologic features of gluten sensitivity in children. *J Pediatr* 2013; Nov 16. pii: S0022-3476(13)01235-3. doi:10.1016/j. jpeds. 2013.10.007.

[50] Biesiekierski JR; Peters SL; Newnham ED; Rosella O; Muir JG; Gibson PR. No effects of gluten in patients with self-reported non-celiac gluten sensitivity after dietary reduction of fermentable, poorly absorbed, short-chain carbohydrates. *Gastroenterology* 2013; 145:320-328.

In: Celiac Disease: An Update
Editors: M. Bozzola, C. Meazza et al.
ISBN: 978-1-63117-088-1
© 2014 Nova Science Publishers, Inc.

Chapter 2

DIAGNOSTIC APPROACH TO SHORT STATURE IN CHILDREN WITH CELIAC DISEASE

Cristina Meazza, Ph.D.[*] *and Mauro Bozzola, M.D.*[†]
[1]Internal Medicine and Therapeutics Department, University of Pavia, Fondazione IRCCS Policlinico San Matteo, Pavia, Italy

ABSTRACT

In recent years, pediatricians have frequently encountered the problem of short stature or stunted growth rate in the context of celiac disease (CD). In fact, the prevalence of CD in patients evaluated for short stature varies between 2% and 10%. The first step in the evaluation of short stature is the exclusion of CD; as many other chronic conditions may be responsible for growth failure, this is followed by an endocrinological investigation and an evaluation of GH secretion. In fact, false GH responses to pharmacological tests have been observed, followed by their normalization after initiation of a gluten-free diet (GFD). Furthermore, after the start of a GFD, catch-up growth is generally observed, and the celiac child usually returns to his/her normal growth curve for weight and height within 1-2 years. The evaluation of GH secretion should be performed in CD children who show no catch-up

---

[*] E-mail: c.meazza@smatteo.pv.it.
[†] E-mail: mauro.bozzola@unipv.it.

growth after at least one year of a strict GFD, and after seronegativity for anti-tissue transglutaminase and anti-endomysial antibodies have been confirmed. In subjects with CD and growth hormone deficiency (GHD), substitutive therapy with GH should be administered at standard doses and should be promptly started, in order to obtain complete catch-up growth. The long-term effects of GH therapy in children who follow a strict GFD are similar to those observed in children with idiopathic GHD.

Finally, the existence of a close relationship between CD and autoimmune diseases, such as thyroid disorders and diabetes mellitus type I, is suggested by the fact that CD is an autoimmune disorder. The pathogenetic mechanism is still not completely known and, only partly, linked to the increase in intestinal permeability.

INTRODUCTION

Recent scientific studies have provided data that extend the diagnostic work-up for celiac disease (CD) to subjects who, even in the absence of gastrointestinal symptoms, show extraintestinal symptoms including short stature and/or delayed puberty.

The prevalence of CD in patients evaluated for short stature varies between 2% and 10%, which exceeds the prevalence for growth hormone deficiency (GHD) and every other endocrine disorder [1-5]. The pathogenesis of short stature associated with CD is not yet completely known, although it has traditionally been attributed to generalized or selective malnutrition, such as zinc malabsorption [6].

AUXOLOGICAL APPROACH

In a child with a stature below the 3rd percentile (figure 1) [Footnotes: the percentile represents the number of subjects of the same age, sex and ethnic group distributed according to percentage of stature, weight, etc.; for example, a child is below the 3rd percentile when, out of a 100 subjects, he/she is among the three shortest] or with growth deceleration (figure 2), a diagnostic work-up should be started to identify any pathological cause.

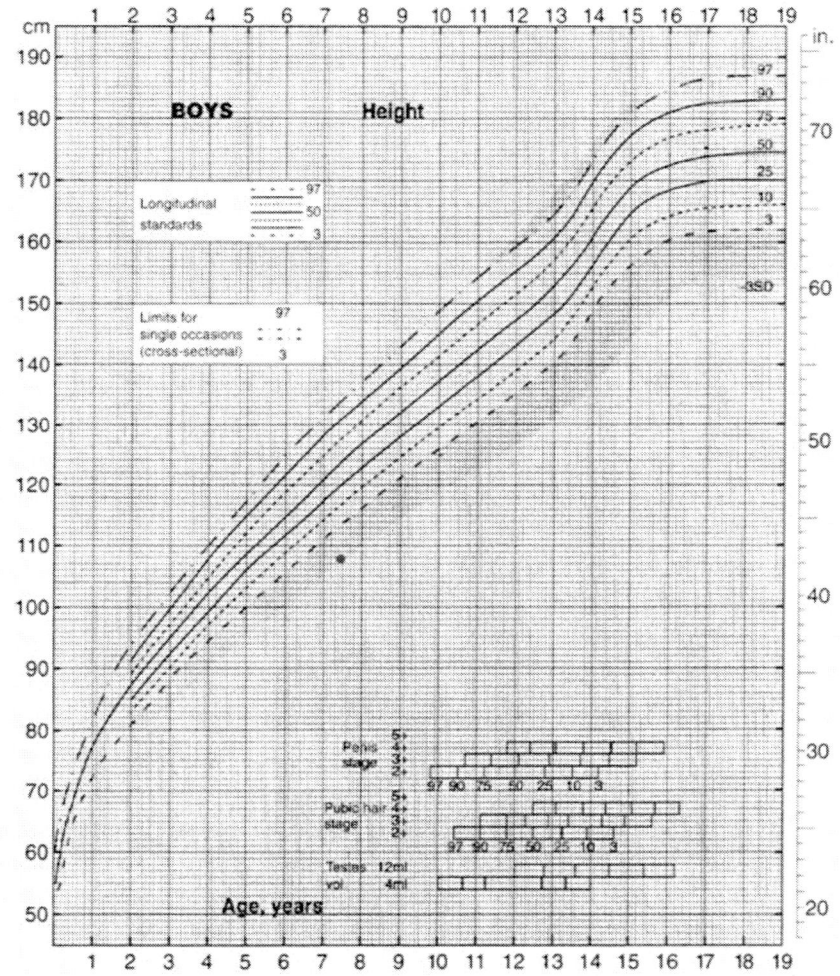

Figure 1. Patient with height below the 3rd percentile.

On the contrary, if a pre-pubertal child shows a stature close to the 3th percentile, but grows along the same percentile (figure 3), an endocrinological evaluation, is not indicated, only an annual growth follow-up.

If, instead, a child grows on a percentile lower than his genetic target or when first pubertal signs (appearance of the mammary gland in female subjects and increased testicular volume in male subjects) are already evident, the diagnostic work-up should be immediately started, without waiting for a growth rate decrease.

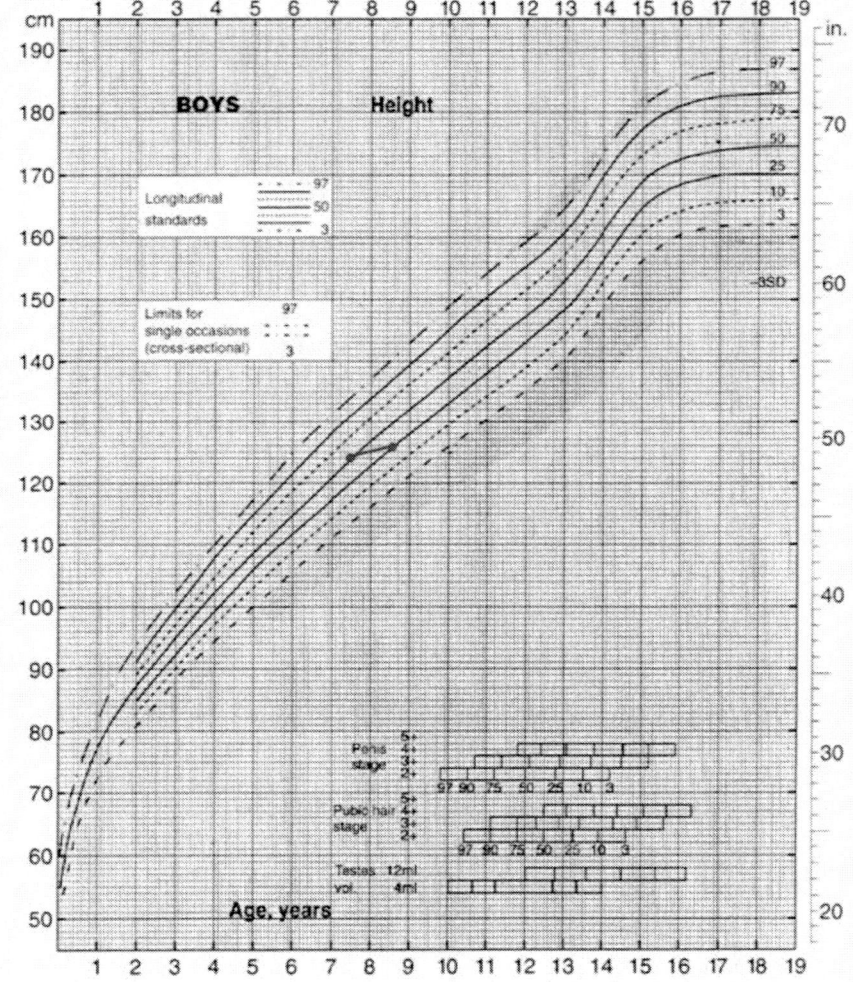

Figure 2. Patient with height, initially above the 50th percentile, that decreases to a lower percentile.

First of all, it is necessary to evaluate whether the short stature is clinically ascribable to a normal variant of the growth pattern (e.g., familial short stature or constitutional delay of growth and puberty) or to a specific pathology (e.g., achondroplasia, hormonal dysfunction). In the differential diagnosis, to discern between familial short stature and/or constitutional delay of growth and puberty and endocrine conditions, a bone age evaluation is useful, since it indicates the subject's growth potential.

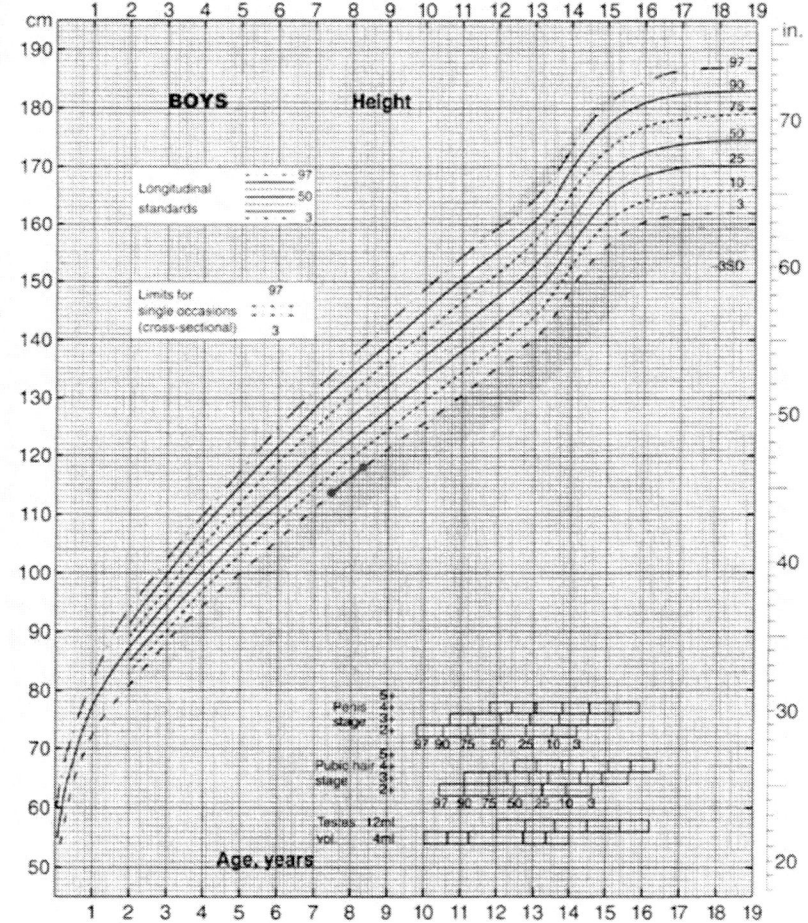

Figure 3. Patient with height within the 3rd percentile that does not decrease to a lower percentile.

Therefore, the next step is the exclusion of other possible conditions responsible for growth failure, including kidney or liver disease, skeletal disorders, subclinical hypothyroidism, intestinal malabsorption, such as

Crohn's disease and CD. It is accepted practice to also exclude the CD, in whom GHD is suspected, before evaluating GH secretion, since false GH responses to pharmacological tests have been observed, followed by their normalization after initiation of a gluten-free diet (GFD). Insulin-like growth factor I (IGF-I), which is considered the peripheral GH mediator, is low in patients with insufficient GH secretion, but is not a discriminating factor for GH secretion, since its level is influenced also by the nutritional status of the subject [7].

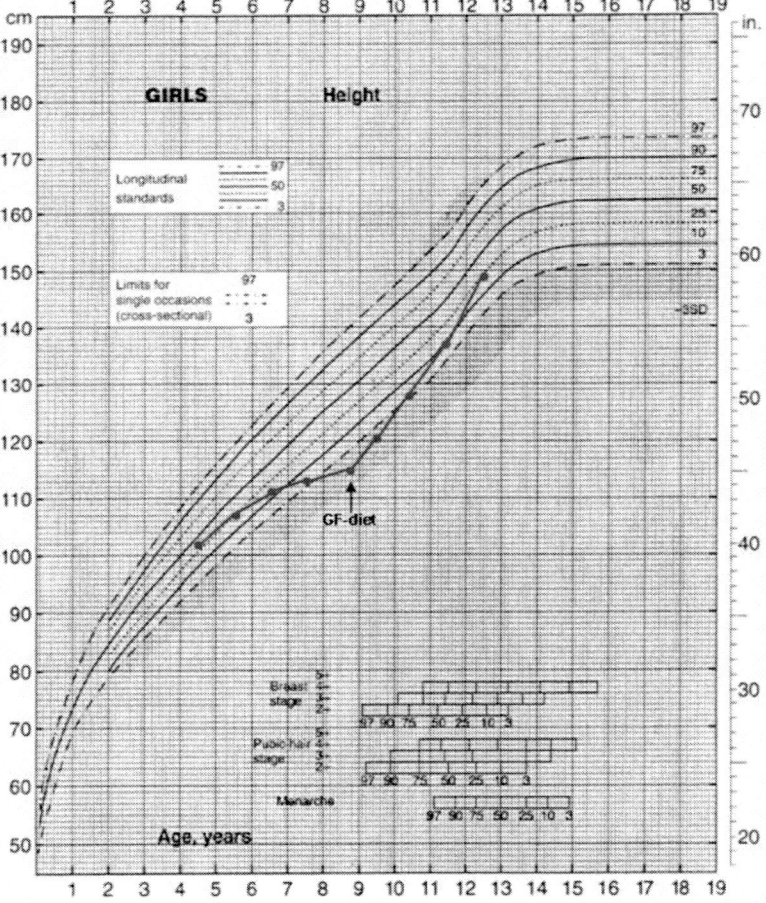

Figure 4. Deceleration of growth rate in a CD child and catch-up growth after the introduction of a GFD.

Furthermore, in a patient with delayed appearance of pubertal signs (such as absence of the mammary gland over 13 years of age in female subjects and >4 ml testicular volume in male subjects over 15 years of age), it is necessary to exclude CD. In fact, after resolution of a pathological condition which may have determined growth deceleration, spontaneous catch-up growth is generally observed (figure 4).

Also in CD, after the start of a GFD, catch-up growth is generally observed and the celiac child usually returns to his/her normal growth curve for weight and height within 1-2 years [6, 8]. Therefore, a careful auxological follow-up is necessary with biannual evaluations to verify growth and weight catch-up, in addition to the annual evaluation of serological negativity. In fact, to confirm dietary compliance the annual monitoring of anti-tTG-IgA is recommended, in consideration of its high sensitivity and specificity. If after 1-2 years of a GFD the subject does not show clear catch-up growth, in the presence of seronegativity for specific celiac antibodies, the evaluation of GH secretion in response to at least two pharmacological stimuli is mandatory [7-9]. It has been observed that 0.23% of children with short stature show an association between CD and GHD [10].

In the presence of a normal GH response to at least one pharmacological stimulus and IGF-I values within the normal range for sex and age, the auxological follow-up should be repeated. In case of a pathological response (i.e., GH peak<10 ng/ml with both stimulus tests) and in the presence of a negative specific serology, once the basal levels of FT4, TSH, ACTH and cortisol have been verified, and poor glucose tolerance after delivery of oral load of glucose has been excluded, substitutive therapy with recombinant human GH should be started as in patients with idiopathic GHD. A nuclear magnetic resonance imaging of the brain is required to exclude any morphological abnormality of the hypothalamic-pituitary region. In the rare cases of GHD associated with a deficiency in one or more pituitary hormones (TSH, ACTH, LH, FSH, ADH), correct hormonal secretion should be restored by substitutive therapy with the missing hormones before starting GH treatment. A deficit in pituitary gonadotropins, LH and FSH, may be assessed only during puberty when in normal children a pubertal gonadotropin increase occurs.

Rarely, reduced GH biological activity may be suspected, on the basis of conflicting results: a normal GH response to pharmacological tests and low IGF-I levels (<2 standard deviations below average), in the presence of normal nutritional status and thyroid function (FT4 e TSH). If the IGF-I generation test shows a normalization of low somatomedin levels after four exogenous subcutaneous GH administrations (0.025 mg/Kg per day), the possibility of starting GH treatment should be considered.

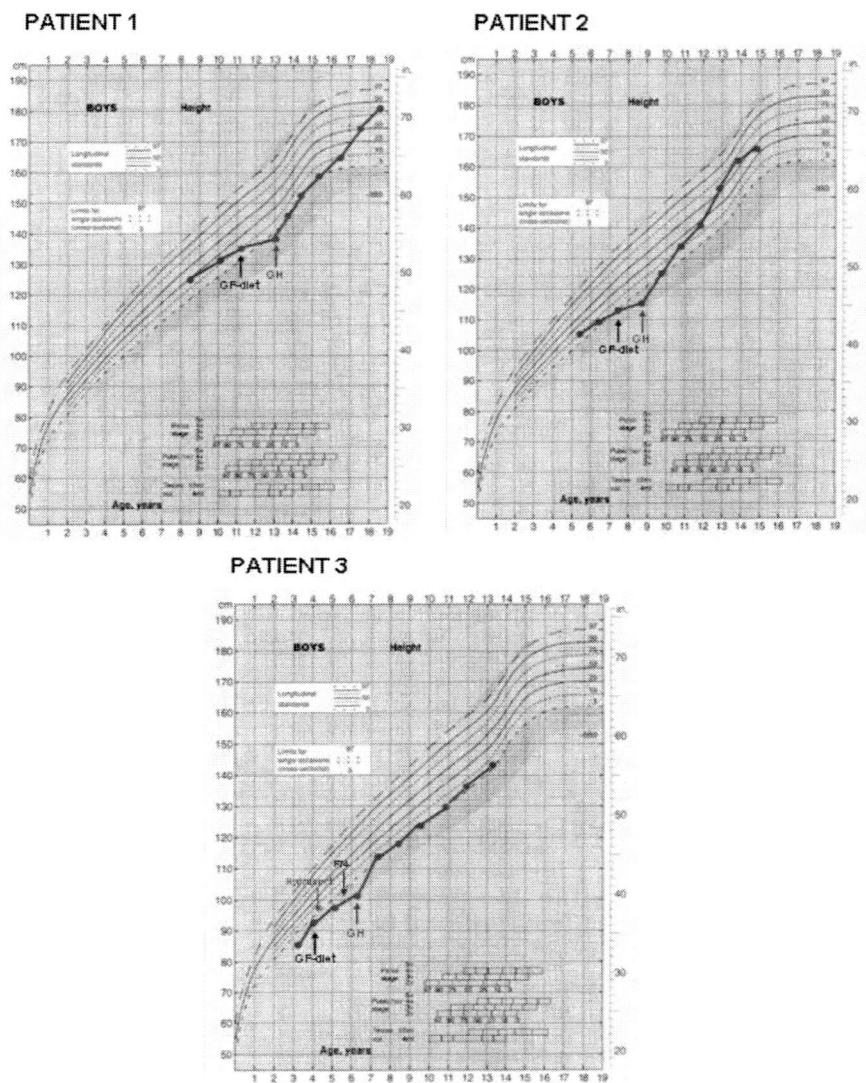

Figure 5. Celiac disease and isolated GHD in patients 1 and 2 and multiple deficiencies in patient 3. Patient 3 is still in treatment with substitutive hormones.

Celiac patients with GHD should be treated with the same GH dosage as patients with idiopathic GHD (0.25 mg/kg/week s.c.), administered in the evening before sleeping to mime the physiological nighttime elevation of the hormone. In the case of associated hormonal deficiencies, the dose of levothyroxine, hydrocortisone, estradiol, testosterone enantate and desmopressin are the same one used in patients without CD. In celiac patients with GHD, the response to substitutive treatment is similar to that of subjects with idiopathic GHD.

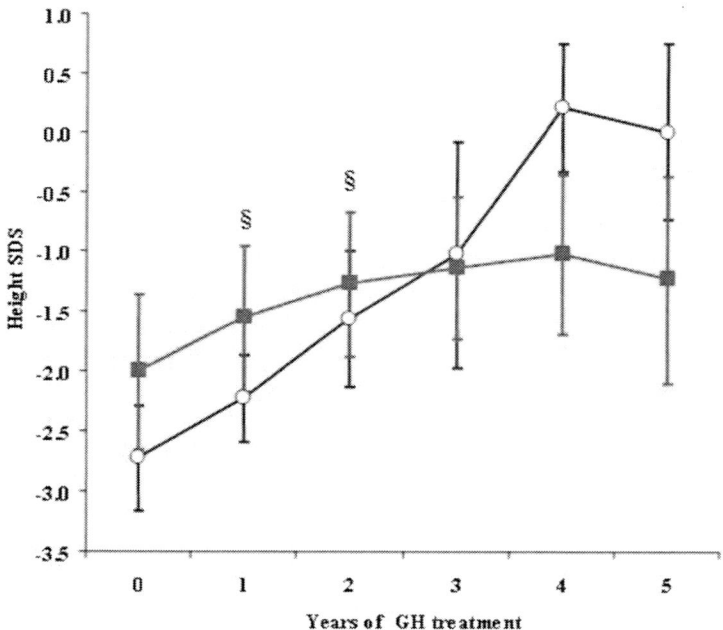

Figure 6. Height before and during the first 5 years of substitutive GH therapy in CD patients with GHD (blue line) and in patients with idiopathic GHD (red line). The data are expressed as the mean and standard deviation.
§ $p<0.05$ time 1 versus time 0 and time 2 versus time 1 for the corresponding group (t-test for paired samples).

Our recent study was the first to clearly demonstrate reduced GH secretion in three pre-pubertal children with CD who showed no catch-up growth after 12 months of a strict GFD in spite of seronegativity for celiac antibodies [8]. Therefore, in these patients GH deficiency was demonstrated based on clinical parameters including short stature, growth deceleration, delayed bone age and GH peak <10 ng/ml during at least two pharmacological stimulus tests [11]. The coexistence of other hormone deficiencies including thyroid function (FT4 e TSH) and adrenal function (circulating cortisol) were also reported. Substitutive GH therapy was therefore started at the recommended weekly dosage of 0.25 mg/kg subdivided in 6 daily subcutaneous doses as in patients with isolated idiopathic GHD, while hydrocortisone and levothyroxine were administered in the subject with multiple deficit as in multiple GHD patients. Both height and growth velocity significantly improved during the therapy confirming that the absence of catch-up growth after a GFD was not due to malnutrition, but to low GH secretion. The growth rate increased especially during the first year of GH therapy and then tapered, however it always remained above pre-treatment values [8] (figure 5).

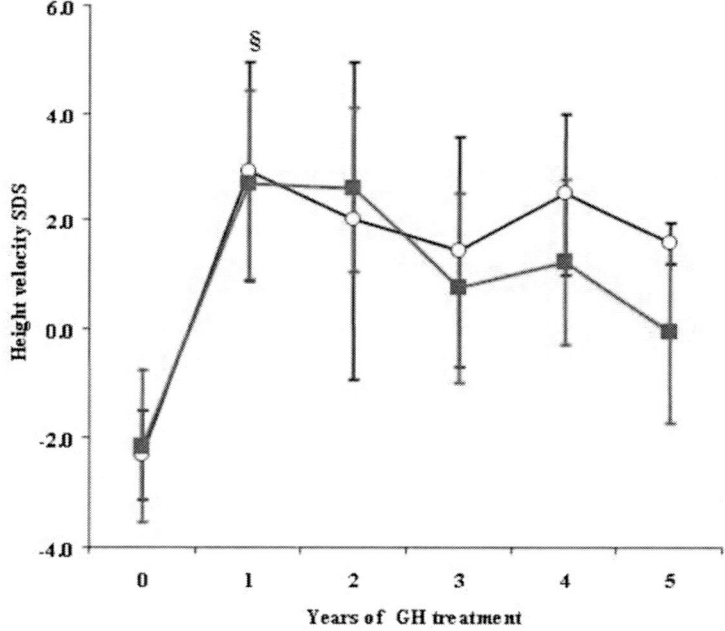

Figure 7. Growth rate before and during the first 5 years of substitutive GH therapy in patients with CD and GHD (blue line) and in patients with idiopathic GHD (red line). The data are expressed as the mean and standard deviation.
§ p<0.05 time 1 versus time 0 for the corresponding group (t-test for paired samples).

In a subsequent study, conducted in ten pre-pubertal children with CD and GHD, and compared with a group of children of the same age with idiopathic GHD treated for five years with the same GH dosages, a similar increase in height and growth velocity was noted [12] (figures 6 and 7).

The growth velocity for patients of both groups increased significantly during the first year of therapy ($p<0.005$) and, subsequently remained constant, but always above the pre-treatment values. During the fourth year of therapy the growth velocity of children with CD and GHD was higher than that of children with only idiopathic GHD.

For some subjects in this study the growth velocity was followed until attainment of final adult height (growth velocity was< 2 cm/year at the time of the last examination). This stature, considered "near final height", did not differ in the two groups (CD patients with GHD: 0.05±0.56 SDS; patients with idiopathic GHD: -0.73±0.81 SDS, p=0.154) (figure 8).

Compliance is very important in order to obtain a good response to GH therapy. Clinical results suggest, in fact, that CD patients with GHD do not respond to hormonal substitutive therapy if they do not observe a strict GFD.

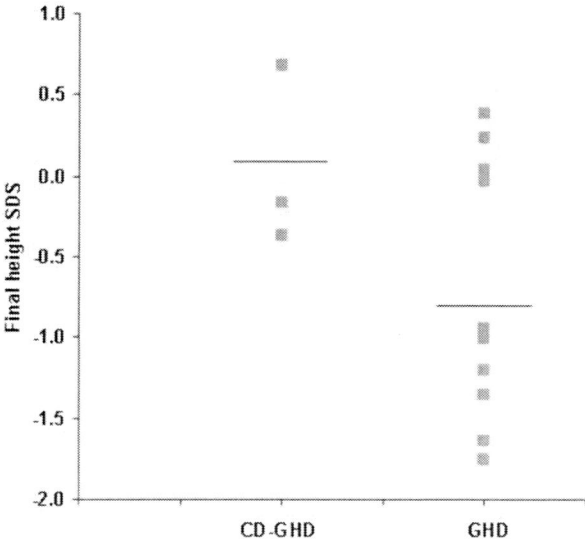

Figure 8. Final height of CD patients with GHD (left) and those with idiopathic GHD (right). The horizontal lines represent the mean value.

DEVELOPMENT OF AUTOIMMUNE CONDITIONS IN CHILDREN WITH CD

The existence of a close relationship between CD and autoimmune diseases is suggested by the fact that CD is an autoimmune disorder. The pathogenetic mechanism is still not completely known and, has been only partly linked to an increase in intestinal permeability, which allows the passage of macromolecules. Furthermore, in CD patients the increased risk of developing other autoimmune diseases seems to be related to the duration of gluten exposure which can be the trigger in genetically-predisposed individuals.

The frequent association of CD with other autoimmune thyroid disorders is based on shared immunopathological mechanisms linked to the haplotype HLA-B8 and -DR3, which are more frequent in these patients compared with the general population. The prevalence varies from 4% to 14% and the most frequent association is between CD and Hashimoto thyroiditis. Furthermore, in the absence of alterations in thyroid function, echographic alterations and increased anti-thyroid peroxidase antibodies have more frequently been observed in CD patients compared with the healthy population. Therefore, in CD subjects it is necessary to periodically monitor thyroid function (FT4 and TSH) and autoantibodies (anti-thyroid thyroglobulin antibodies (anti-TG) and anti-thyroid peroxidase antibodies (anti-TPO), in the case of a TSH increase.

In the presence of anti-thyroid antibodies, if Hashimoto thyroiditis is suspected, a thyroid echography should be performed to evaluate the structure of the thyroid parenchyma. In the rare case of reduced FT4 and increased TSH, low-dosage treatment with levothyroxine (12.5-25 µg per day, to be taken orally at least 30 minutes before breakfast) should be started, and increased to the full dosage in 1-2 months, with biannual monitoring FT4 and TSH, without considering anti-TPO and anti-TG levels.

Another widely documented association is that between CD and type 1 diabetes mellitus (T1DM). Genetic studies report a higher frequency of HLA-B8,-DR3 and -DQW2 both in patients with T1DM and in those with CD in comparison with the general population. Furthermore, alterations in β cells and enterocytes seems to be due to the same factors, such as proinflammatory cytokines (e.g., interferon-γ and TNF-α). In most cases

CD is diagnosed months or years after the onset of T1DM and the probability of developing CD increases with the duration of diabetes. Predictive parameters of the risk to develop T1DM include the presence of anti-insulin antibodies (IA2), anti-glutammic acid decarboxylase antibodies (GAD), anti-zinc transporter 8 antibodies (ZnT8). It is common practice to evaluate at the onset of T1DM, and annually, thereafter CD serology and, in case of abnormal anti-tTG levels, a duodenal-jejunal biopsy is required to evidence any intestinal damage suggestive of CD.

In cases of potential CD, when a positive serological test does not correspond with any histological intestinal mucosal alterations (stage Marsh 0 or Marsh 1), an annual auxo-endocrinological and serological follow-up are recommended.

Adherence to a strict GFD favors regular growth, prevents CD complications as well as the onset of other autoimmune diseases.

TAKE HOME MESSAGES

1. The evaluation of GH secretion should be performed in CD children who show no catch-up growth after at least one year on a strict GFD, after seronegativity of anti-tissue transglutaminase and anti-endomysial antibodies has been confirmed.
2. In subjects with CD and GHD, substitutive therapy with GH should be administered at standard doses and should be promptly started, in order to obtain complete catch-up growth.
3. The long-term effects of GH therapy in children who follow a strict GFD are similar to those observed in children with idiopathic GHD.
4. During follow-up, it is important to verify compliance with the diet and to check the specific serology, auxological parameters, thyroid function, cortisol values and glyco-metabolic profile.

CONCLUSION

In the case of a child with a documented CD diagnosis it is necessary:

1. to carefully assess stature and note the growth chart percentile, comparing it with the genetic target;
2. to evaluate pubertal development;
3. to calculate growth velocity retrospectively or by means of a new distance measurement at least six months later. Normal growth velocity does not require further endocrinological investigation;
4. to perform screening examinations, in case of growth velocity deceleration (<25th percentile), to exclude reduced thyroid function and organ disease. If these parameters are normal, the next step is the evaluation of GH secretion in response to a first pharmacological stimulus followed by a second in case of GH peak <10 ng/ml. In peripubertal patients, the pharmacological stimulus response may be retested after priming with steroid treatment, to exclude false GHD. Children with both GH peaks <10 ng/ml should begin GH substitutive therapy after the glyco-metabolic profile evaluation, to exclude altered glucose tolerance. A brain magnetic resonance may be required to rule out morphological hypothalamus-pituitary region anomalies. In case of total deficit (GH peaks <5 ng/ml), possible deficits in other pituitary hormones, such as ACTH, TSH, FSH, LH should be investigated. These may also be investigated after starting GH therapy.

Once GHD has been excluded, IGF-I dosage under basal conditions may be evaluated. If the value is <2 standard deviations below average, it may be useful to perform an "IGF-I generation test" to evaluate reduced GH bioactivity. If the IGF-I value does not increase after GH administration, a GH insensitivity evaluation may be performed. In the presence of typical syndromic features, it may be useful to perform a karyotype, since CD is frequently associated with chromosomal abnormalities, such as Down syndrome and Turner syndrome.

CLINICAL EVALUATION

Auxological Evaluation

The pediatrician should carefully evaluates the child's height using precise methods of measurement and suitable tools such as a stadiometer and an infantometer (the latter for children less than 2 years of age, who are measured while lying down) (figure 9).

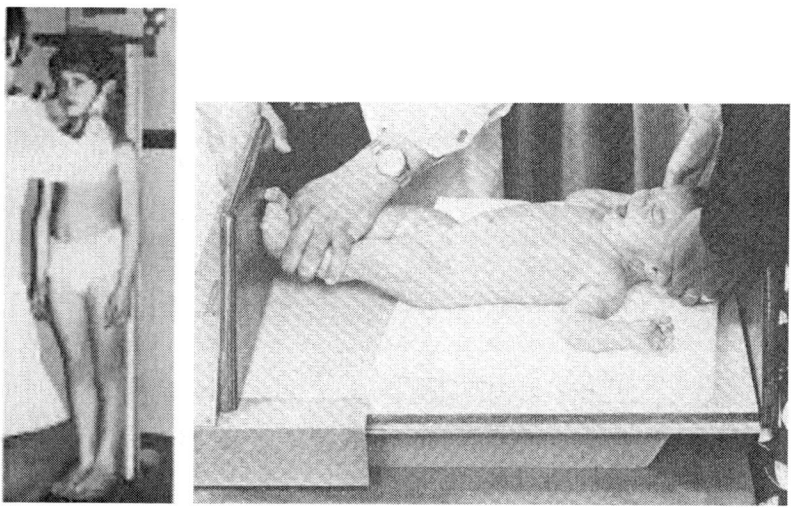

Figure 9. Measurement of height and length with, respectively, Harpenden stadiometer (left) and Harpenden infantometer (right).

Growth percentile can be determined by correlating the child's height with his chronological age on a growth chart, specific for males and females, highlighting possible deviations from the norm. International (Tanner) and national (Cacciari) growth charts report the normal population growth rate from birth to adult age (figure 10).

Growth deceleration can be highlighted by calculating the difference between two measurements, at least 6-12 months apart, using suitable Tanner percentile charts, specific for males and females (figure 11). A height velocity below the 25th percentile or above the 75th percentile may require close diagnostic examination.

Weight evaluation with body mass index calculation (BMI), must be included in the assessment of height and growth velocity, in order to detect overweight or underweight subjects.

Upon completion of the auxological exam, genetic target [(formula to calculate the genetic target (father's height + mother's height)/2) + 6.5 if male or -6.5 if female)] and pubertal development should be evaluated.

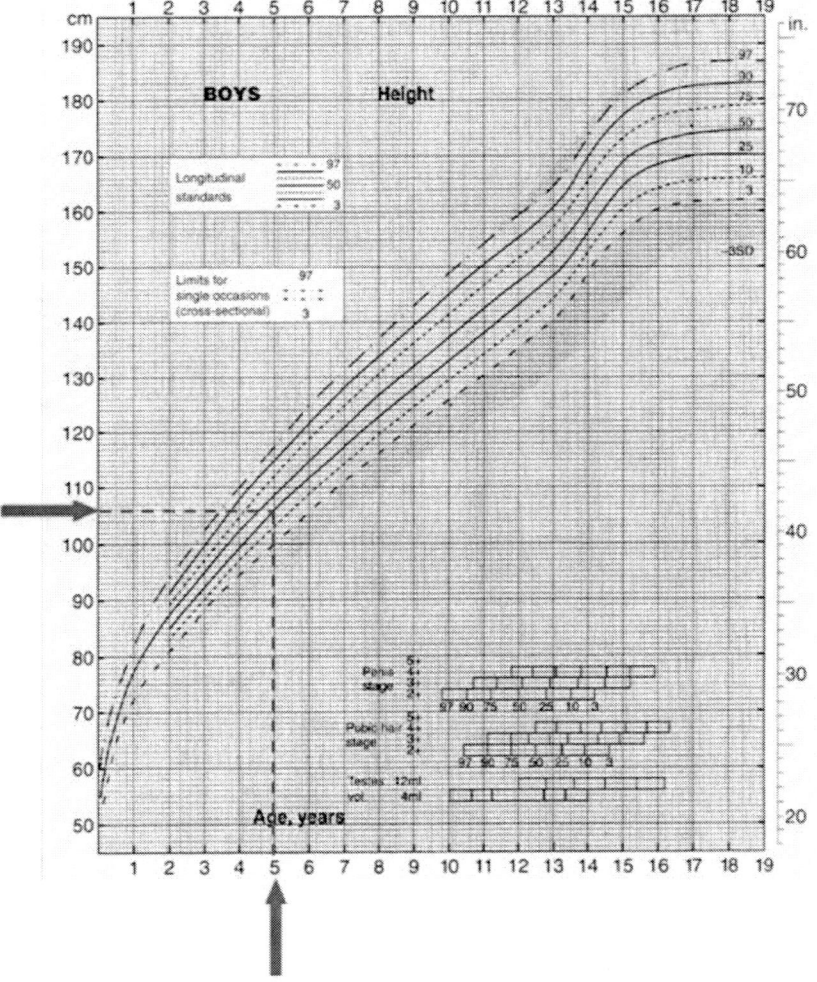

Figure 10. Interpolation of age and height values on a growth chart to detect the percentile.

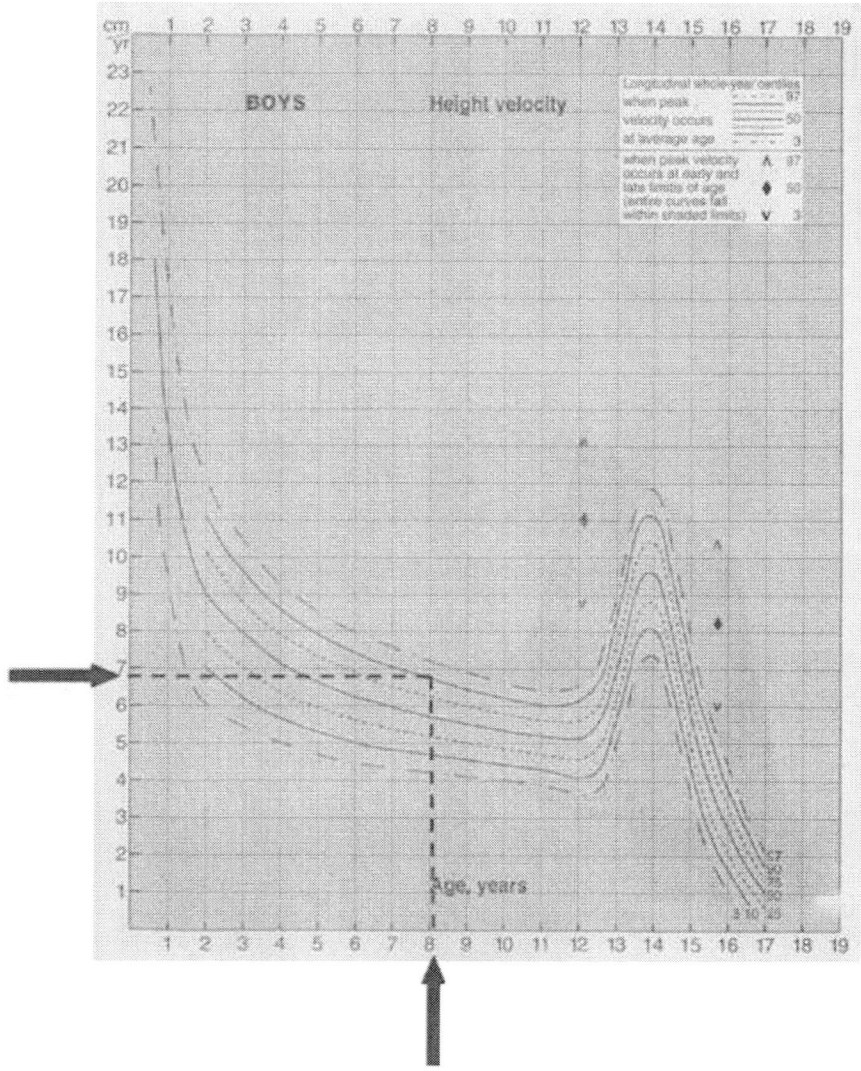

Figure 11. Interpolation of age and height velocity values on a growth chart to detect the percentile.

Pubertal development is divided into five stages, evaluated, depending on male or female, according to pubic hair (PH), breast development (B) and male genitalia morphology (G). Testicular volume is quantified using a

Prader orchidometer and compared with the suitable percentiles to verify normal development (figure 12).

In case of advanced puberty (appearance of menarche in females and adult testicular volume in males), the pubertal spurt could already have reached its peak, as evidenced by x-ray scans showing the closure of cartilage growth.

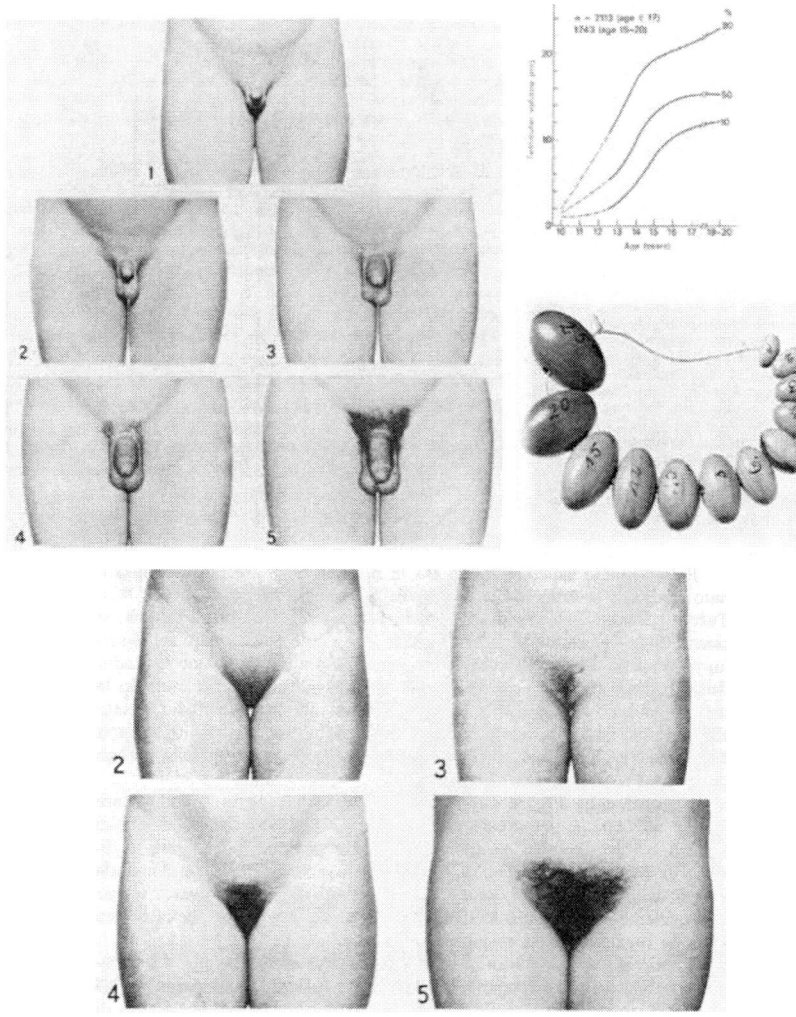

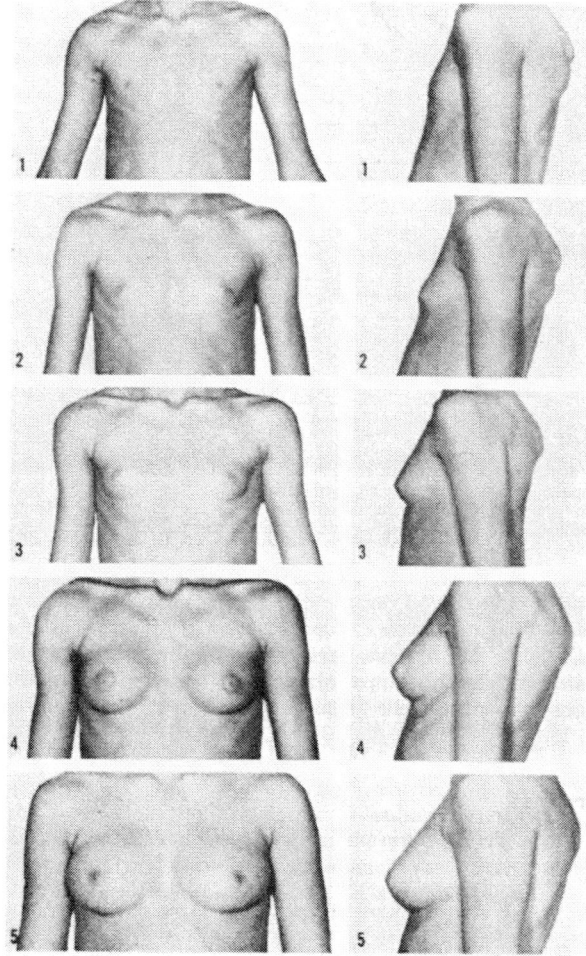

Figure 12. Pubertal development stages in male and female, Prader orchidometer

Bone Age

Bone age is evaluated with an x-ray scan of the left hand and is assessed using the Greulich and Pyle radiological atlas [13]. This is the most-commonly used method for rapid evaluation. It takes into consideration the number and the dimensions of the hand and wrist bones. Bone age can also be assessed using the Tanner and Whitehouse method in which a score is given to each bone (skeletal maturation stage) and the measurements are noted on a percentile chart [14]. In this case, it is important to highlight that bone age evaluation depends on the operator's expertise. In a normal child, bone age can match chronological age or may be slightly delayed.

GH Deficiency [15, 16]

In current clinical practice, the diagnosis of GHD relies on biochemical measurement of GH secretion after two stimulation tests, notwithstanding their lack of precision. Different commercially available assays for measuring GH exist and several studies have shown an inter-assay variability for GH values which leads to a wide discrepancy in the results obtained in different laboratories. For correct evaluation of test results it is necessary to take into consideration standard references and consider the laboratory assay methodology. However, it is still common in clinical practice to use the traditional cut-off value of 10 ng/ml. The consensus guidelines of the Growth Hormone Research Society for diagnosis of GHD in children have established that, in a child with suspected isolated GHD, two stimulation tests are required. The second test is needed due to the widespread presence of first false pathological tests (20% of subjects). On the contrary, in a child with central nervous system pathology or cranial irradiation only one GH stimulation test is needed. Many different stimuli are currently used to induce GH secretion, since they act through different mechanisms.

The first stimulus generally used is arginine. This is administered intravenously (0.5 g/kg of a 10% solution) over a 30-min period and, in case of a GH peak <10 ng/ml, is followed by an insulin test (0.1 U/kg i.v.), clonidine test (0.15 mg/m^2 p.o.) or glucagon test (0.03 mg/kg i.m. or s.c.), depending on the center's expertise. Two GH concentration peaks of less than 5 ng/ml are necessary to define severe GHD and at least one peak between 5 and 10 ng/ml indicates partial GHD. Since sex steroids cause an increase in GH secretion during puberty, priming with sex steroids (for example estradiol or testosterone for three days, depending on gender) before the GH stimulation test may facilitate GH release in peripubertal children.

Overweight children should be evaluated after a suitable restrictive diet, since they can have a falsely reduced GH response to pathological tests. At the discretion of the center, a GHRH plus arginine test may also be employed. The cut-off for this test is considered 20 ng/ml for the GH peak. In any case, even in the presence of two positive pathological tests, the diagnosis of GH deficiency cannot be considered absolute in the absence of unequivocal auxological parameters. As recommended by the Growth Hormone Research Society, patients with proven GHD should be treated with GH as soon as possible after the diagnosis is made, in order to obtain normalization of height during childhood and normal adult height [11].

In children treated early, catch-up growth is excellent, although it may be affected by variables such as birth-weight, parents' height, age at start of treatment, extent of the GHD, duration of treatment, height at start of treatment and start of puberty. Growth hormone treatment in childhood can also normalize body composition, reduce body fat, generate a reversible insulin insensitivity, increase the ratio of high-density lipoprotein-total cholesterol, accelerate bone remodeling and increasing bone mineral mass. Growth hormone therapy is administered subcutaneously in the evening and the dose is expressed in mg/kg/day. The recommended daily dose is 0.025-0.05 mg/kg/day for six days a week. In overweight patients it is preferable to calculate the dosage depending on body surface (0.67 mg/m^2/day). Protocols suggest to increase the dosage to 0.03-0.07 mg/kg/day and to administer therapy every day (without a weekly rest) during puberty to maximize growth during this period of life.

Subcutaneous administration is the standard delivery procedure due to its simplicity of execution and good patient compliance. It is necessary, however, to vary the site of inoculation to avoid lypodistrophy which may prevent GH absorption. If adequately motivated and instructed, the child's family will administer the GH therapy with care and regularity.

GH treatment should be monitored, evaluating biannually the biochemical markers of thyroid function (FT4 and TSH) and adrenal function (cortisol levels) and the glyco-metabolic profile (blood glucose, glycated hemoglobin, insulin levels).

Recently in an international study, the importance of IGF-I monitoring in children with GHD was evaluated. The authors concluded that IGF-I monitoring, during GH therapy, is an useful instrument to evaluate treatment adherence and may help clinicians modify the GH dosage to optimize growth. If catch-up growth does not occur, it is opportune to suspend treatment and reconsider the diagnosis. In case of scarce treatment response, chronic associated diseases, anti-GH antibodies (however, exceptional in clinical practice) or concomitant osteocondrodysplasia should be excluded. Patients that suspend substitutive therapy should be followed long term for the risk of negative complications (e.g., bone mass loss). Before deciding whether to suspend or continue GH therapy in a patient who has reached definitive stature and pubertal development, hormonal secretion retesting is needed in order to identify patients at risk of developing adult GH deficiency syndrome.

GH Therapy Side Effects

GH therapy side effects evaluated in the last 20 years have shown a very low incidence. They include benign intracranial hypertension (frequency 1/10,000-1/1,000) paresthesias (frequency 1/1,000-1/100) arthralgias and myalgias (frequency 1/100-1/10) and rarely injection site reactions or skin rash. Generally, these events are due to an increased sensitivity to GH physiological effects (e.g., water and sodium retention, increased growth velocity). Proximal femoral epyphysiolysis or Perthes disease and scoliosis (observed more frequently during puberty) have rarely been described. In case of side effects, reduction or temporary suspension of GH therapy, is recommended. Growth hormone treatment may represent a risk factor for type 2 diabetes mellitus in predisposed subjects (frequency 1/10,000-1/1,000). Among the metabolic effects of therapy, glyco-metabolic unbalance, has always been the most frequent, but this is reversible, while insulin resistance due to treatment is particularly frequent in pubertal age. Furthermore, a biannual glycated hemoglobin evaluation is mandatory in all patients. In the past, GH therapy has been suggested to increase the risk of leukemia or other tumors. However, numerous studies have shown that the incidence of leukemia or other tumors, in patients following long-term GH therapy is not significantly different from the incidence estimated in children without substitutive therapy (1/10,000). Finally, there is no clinical evidence that therapy should be stopped during recurrent disease (e.g., influenza).

Stimulation Tests to Evaluate GH Secretion

Many different stimuli are currently used to induce GH secretion, since they act through different mechanisms. In fact, no stimulation test is completely reliable, although for clinical practice, the insulin-tolerance test (ITT) is the gold standard. Owing to the lack of reproducibility and accuracy of these tests, the clinician should remember that the diagnosis of GHD is mainly based on clinical and auxological findings, and that the results of the stimulation tests are only confirmatory. Stimulation tests include different pharmacological stimuli, as summarized in Table 1.

Table 1. Growth hormone stimulation tests

Stimulus	Dosage	Sampling times (minutes)
Insulin (ITT) i.v.	0.05-0.1 U/Kg	0, 15, 30, 45, 60 and 90
Arginine HCl i.v.	0.5 g/Kg (max 40 g)	0, 30, 60, 90 and 120
L-Dopa p.o.	10 mg/Kg (max 500 mg)	0, 30, 60, 90 and 120
Clonidine i.v.	0.15 mg/m^2	0, 30, 60 and 90
Glucagon i.m.	0.03 mg/Kg (max 1 mg)	0, 60, 120, 150 and 180
GHRH i.v.	1 µg/Kg	0, 15, 30, 45, 60, 90 and 120

i.v.: intravenously; i.m.: intramuscularly; p.o.: per os.

These tests should be performed in pediatric endocrinology centers and patients should be monitored carefully by an experienced team. Although ITT is considered the best stimulation test, it is risky and must be performed with appropriate surveillance. The mechanism of stimulation is a counter-regulatory response to insulin-induced hypoglycemia. To perform the test, 0.1 unit/kg of insulin is administered intravenously in children over 4 years of age and 0.05 unit/kg in younger children. Blood samples for GH analysis and glucose levels should be obtained at 0, 30, 60, 90 and 120 min after administering the insulin dose. At the same times glucose and cortisol levels are also evaluated. The test is considered valid if the blood glucose level decreases by 40-50% of the initial value or reaches less than 40 mg/dl. The GH peak occurs 15-30 min after the glucose nadir.

Arginine stimulates GH secretion by inhibiting somatostatin release through β-adrenergic receptors. Arginine HCl (0.5 g/kg to a maximum of 40 g) is administered intravenously over a 30-min period. Blood samples for GH determination should be taken at 0, 30, 60, 90, 120 min. At the same times insulin levels are also evaluated. The maximum GH peak is expected to occur at 60 min after starting the arginine infusion. Nausea and vomiting are frequently observed side effects.

Clonidine, an α_2-adrenergic agonist, increases GHRH secretion and inhibits somatostatin release. This stimulus is one of the best choices to avoid false-negative results. Clonidine is administered at a dose of 0.15 mg/m^2 (maximum 0.15 mg). Samples for this GH assay should be obtained at 0, 30, 60, 90, 120 and 180 min. Maximal GH secretion is expected at 60 min following clonidine administration and the GH peak is usually greater than the peak response to other tests. Blood pressure should be monitored after clonidine administration as it may fall and, in young children, clonidine causes drowsiness, which may last for several hours.

Glucagon induces GH secretion by stimulating endogenous insulin secretion to compensate for elevated serum glucose levels. It is a good substitute for the ITT, which may be risky in newborns and small children. Glucagon is administered intramuscularly or subcutaneously at a dose of 0.03 mg/kg to a maximum of 1 mg. Serum samples are obtained at 0, 30, 60, 90, 120, 150, 180 min after glucagon administration and the maximal GH peak occurs between 2 and 3 hrs after administering glucagon. At 0, 150, 180 min cortisol levels must be evaluated. During the course of this test, young children may develop nausea and vomiting.

The administration of growth hormone releasing hormone (GHRH) provides data that can directly assess the capacity of the pituitary to secrete GH. Since there is great variability in the GH response owing to fluctuations in somatostatin secretion, and its inhibitors, i.e., pyridostigmine and arginine, these have been used to enhance the GH response and to reduce the intra-and inter-individual variability. The GHRH test, alone or in combination with arginine, is a useful tool to identify defects at the hypothalamic level and is very informative for children with multiple pituitary hormone deficiency. The GHRH plus arginine test is frequently used, since it stimulates GH to a greater extent than the GHRH test alone. GHRH is administered intravenously at a dose of 1 µg/kg (maximum 50 µg) at time 0 and arginine (0.5 g/kg, maximum of 40 g) is administered intravenously from 0-30 minutes. Serum samples for the GH analysis are obtained at -15, 0, 15, 30, 45, 60 and 90 min. The cut-off for this test is considered 20 ng/ml for the GH peak in children while in late adolescent and young adult patients the cut-off for the GH peak is 19 ng/ml. Furthermore, the GHRH plus arginine test is useful for identifying false-positive GHD in children showing a blunted GH response to classic stimuli in contrast with a normal growth rate.

Since sex steroids cause the increase in GH secretion during puberty, priming with sex steroids before the GH stimulation test may facilitate GH release in pre-pubertal children. Priming may be performed with estradiol or ethinylestradiol (a daily dose of 50-100 µg for 3 days) before the GH stimulation test in both boys and girls or 100 mg testosterone depot may be administered between 7 and 10 days before GH stimulation in boys.

The IGFs are GH-dependent peptides that mediate many of the anabolic and mitogenic actions of GH. Since serum levels of IGF-I are stable during the day, it should be possible to assess GH status by measuring IGF-I levels once and, thus, bypass the use of the GH provocation test, with its poor reproducibility. However, IGF-I is not routinely used in the diagnosis of GHD in children because not all the assays for IGF-I show good sensitivity and specificity. Furthermore, IGF-I levels are influenced by age and pubertal development and, although age and puberty-corrected IGF-I reference values have been generated, an overlap between IGF-I values for normal and GHD children still exists, particularly in children younger than 5 years. Moreover, results vary between laboratories because different assay methods are used. Most investigators have used cut-offs of either the fifth percentile or less than -2 SDS to define subnormal levels of IGF-I. Moreover, reduced IGF-I levels may occur in children with malnutrition, hypothyroidism, hepatic disease or diabetes mellitus.

IGFBP-3 levels have also been considered for the detection of GHD. However, no correlation was found between GH levels and serum levels of IGFBP-3 in assessing GHD. In conclusion, although low IGF-I and IGFBP-3 concentrations are suggestive of a diagnosis of severe GHD, normal serum IGF-I and IGFBP-3 values may not allow the exclusion of GHD. Therefore, most authors following the guidelines of the GH Research Society define GHD using stimulation tests [11]. Since they are artificial by nature, pharmacological tests might not always reflect physiological GH secretion. Furthermore, they are expensive and include a significant risk for the patient. Therefore, GH secretion may be evaluated by more physiologic tests with the advantage of minimal side effects for the patient. Although tests such as the exercise test, 24-h GH profiling and urinary GH estimation are no longer used for the diagnosis of GHD in clinical practice, they are still useful for research investigations.

Reduced GH Biological Activity

In addition to a quantitative deficiency, a qualitative GH deficiency may be detected, which results in the presence of GH isoforms with reduced biological activity (Kowarski syndrome). This condition is characterized by a normal response to pharmacological tests with very low IGF-I levels that return to normal after GH administration. The diagnosis is possible thanks to the "IGF-I generation test": the test consists in IGF-I dosing under basal conditions and twelve hours after the last of four daily GH administrations (0.1 IU/kg/day s.c.). Subjects with Kowarski syndrome show a similar phenotype to that of patients with standard GH deficiency, and they respond well to GH substitutive therapy, at least in the first years of treatment.

REFERENCES

[1] Cacciari E; Salardi S; Volta U; Biasco G; Lazzari R; Corazza GR; Feliciani M; Cicognani A; Partesotti S; Azzaroni D; et al. Can antigliadin antibody detect symptomless coeliac disease in children with short stature? *Lancet* 1985 29; 1: 1469-1471.

[2] Hill ID; Dirks MH; Liptak GS; Colletti RB; Fasano A; Guandalini S; Hoffenberg EJ; Horvath K; Murray JA; Pivor M; Seidman EG; North American Society for Pediatric Gastroenterology, Hepatology and Nutrition. Guideline for the diagnosis and treatment of celiac disease in children: recommendations of the North American Society for Pediatric Gastroenterology, Hepatology and Nutrition. *J Pediatr Gastroenterol Nutr* 2005; 40: 1-19.

[3] Rosenbach Y; Dinari G; Zahavi I; Nitzan M. Short stature as the major manifestation of coeliac disease in older children. *Clin Pediatr (Phila)* 1986; 25: 13-16.

[4] Stenhammar L; Fallstrom SP; Jansson ; Jansson U; Lindberg T. Coeliac disease in children with short stature without gastrointestinal symptoms. *Eur J Pediatr* 1986; 145: 185-186.
[5] Bonamico M; Scirè G; Mariani P; Pasquino AM; Triglione P; Scaccia S; Ballati G; Boscherini B. Short stature as the primary manifestation of monosymptomatic celiac disease. *J Pediatr Gastroenterol Nutr* 1992; 14: 12-16.
[6] Knudtzon J; Fluge G; Aksnes L. Routine measurements of gluten antibodies in children of short stature. *J Pediatr Gastroenterol Nutr* 1991; 12: 190-194.
[7] Bianchi C; Busetto F; Sterpa A; Buonomo A. Deficit transitorio di GH in corso di morbo celiaco. *Min Ped* 1980; 32: 891-897.
[8] Bozzola M; Giovenale D; Bozzola E; Meazza C; Martinetti M; Tinelli C; Corazza GR. Growth hormone deficiency and coeliac disease: an unusual association? *Clin Endocrinol* 2005; 62: 372-375.
[9] Karlberg J; Henter JI; Tassin E; Lindblad BS. Longitudinal analysis of infantile growth in children with celiac disease. *Acta Paediatr Scand* 1988; 77: 516-524.
[10] Giovenale D; Meazza C; Cardinale GM; Sposito M; Mastrangelo C; Messini B; Citro G; Delvecchio M; Di Maio S; Bozzola M. The prevalence of growth hormone deficiency and celiac disease in short children. *Clin Med Res* 2006; 4: 180-183.
[11] Growth Hormone Research Society. Consensus guidelines for the diagnosis and treatment of growth hormone (GH) deficiency in childhood and adolescence: summary statement of the GH Research Society. GH Research Society. *J Clin Endocrinol Metab* 2000; 85: 3990-3993.
[12] Giovenale D; Meazza C; Cardinale GM; Farinelli E; Mastrangelo C; Messini B; Citro G; Delvecchio M; Di Maio S; Possenti I; Bozzola M. Treatment with growth hormone (GH) in prepubertal coeliac children with GH deficiency. *J Pediatr Gastroenterol Nutr* 2007; 45: 433-437.
[13] Greulich WW; Pyle SI. *Radiographic atlas of skeletal development of the hand and wrist,* 2nd ed. Stanford, CA: Stanford University Press; 1959.
[14] Tanner JM; Whitehouse RH; Cameron N; Marshall WA; Healy MJR; Godstein H. Assessment of skeletal maturation and prediction

of adult height (TW2 Method). New York USA: Academic Press; 1983.

[15] Bozzola M; Meazza C. Growth hormone deficiency: diagnosis and therapy in children. *Expert Rev Endocrinol Metab* 2010, 5: 273-284.

[16] Bozzola M; Meazza C. *Il deficit di GH in età pediatrica.* Salerno, Italia: Momento Medico; 2012.

INDEX

A

achondroplasia, 53
acid, 13, 61
ACTH, 55, 62
ADH, 55
adhesion, 30
adults, 19, 21, 25, 26, 36
Africa, 6
age, 2, 8, 12, 13, 20, 23, 31, 41, 50, 53, 55, 58, 59, 63, 64, 65, 67, 69, 70, 71, 73
agonist, 72
algorithm, 28, 29
allergy, 2, 41
alopecia, 16
anaphylaxis, 41
anemia, 13, 14, 16, 17, 18
antibody, 5, 21, 30, 31, 32, 35, 39, 48, 74
antiepileptic drugs, 20
antigen, 2, 8, 9, 10, 28, 29, 30
antigen-presenting cells, 8, 30
apoptosis, 27
appetite, 13
arginine, 68, 69, 72
arginine test, 69, 72
arthritis, 35, 36
assessment, 25, 64
asthma, 41
asymptomatic, 13, 22, 24, 25, 27, 29, 39

ataxia, 20, 21, 45
atrophy, 5, 11, 15, 21, 23, 30, 33, 34, 37
autoantibodies, 10, 11, 19, 20, 21, 22, 25, 30, 38, 39, 45, 47, 60
autoimmune diseases, vii, 3, 10, 26, 31, 35, 50, 60, 61
autoimmune hepatitis, 26, 27, 29, 47
autoimmunity, 17

B

base, 22, 45, 46
benign, 40, 70
biliary cirrhosis, 17, 24, 26
biological activity, 55, 74
biomarkers, 42
biopsy, 4, 5, 11, 18, 22, 23, 25, 32, 33, 35, 43, 45, 61
birth weight, 22
bleeding, 18
blood, 22, 23, 24, 31, 69, 71
body composition, 69
body fat, 69
body mass index (BMI), 38, 64
bone, 19, 38, 53, 58, 67, 69, 70
bone age, 53, 58, 68
bone mass, 70
bones, 27, 67
bowel, 4, 13, 32, 33, 36, 37, 42

Index

C

brain, 55, 62
breastfeeding, 9, 10, 22
breeding, 39

calcifications, 14, 17, 20, 45
calcium, 19, 30
cancer, 16, 18
capsule, 33
carbohydrates, 42, 48
carcinoma, 24
cardiac muscle, 22
cardiomyopathy, 17, 22, 45
cartilage, 66
causal relationship, 16, 18, 22
celiac disease, v, vii, viii, 1, 2, 3, 26, 29, 44, 49
celiac patient, 3, 6, 8, 11, 14, 16, 18, 19, 20, 21, 25, 26, 27, 28, 40, 57
central nervous system, 27, 68
cerebellum, 21
children, vii, 15, 18, 21, 22, 25, 26, 31, 32, 33, 36, 38, 39, 42, 43, 44, 48, 49, 55, 57, 59, 61, 63, 68, 69, 70, 71, 72, 73, 74, 75, 76
China, 6
cholangitis, 24, 26
cholesterol, 69
chromosomal abnormalities, 62
chromosome, 8
cirrhosis, 17, 24, 25
classification, 33, 34, 35
clinical presentation, 12, 37, 44
clinical trials, 39
colitis, 36
colon, 36
compliance, 22, 32, 38, 40, 45, 55, 61, 69
complications, 11, 15, 19, 36, 61, 70
computed tomography, 20
consumption, 39, 43
contamination, 38, 39
control group, 26
cortisol, 55, 58, 61, 69, 71, 72
cost, 31, 32, 37

cytokines, 9, 10, 60
cytolytic activity, 11
cytomegalovirus, 37
cytometry, 15

D

damages, 27
defects, 13, 14, 72
deficiency(ies), 8, 13, 14, 16, 17, 18, 31, 32, 36, 37, 42, 44, 50, 55, 56, 57, 58, 69, 70, 72, 74, 75, 76
deficit, 55, 58, 62, 76
dehydration, 41
deposition, 30
deposits, 21, 23, 28, 30, 35, 48
derivatives, 5
dermatitis herpetiformis, 13, 16, 18
detection, 15, 31, 35, 73
detoxification, 40
developing countries, 7
deviation, 57, 58
diabetes, 8, 17, 42, 45, 50, 61, 70, 73
diagnostic criteria, 4, 47
diarrhea, 2, 12, 13, 16, 41, 42
diet, vii, 1, 2, 4, 5, 6, 7, 12, 13, 15, 16, 18, 19, 22, 28, 29, 30, 38, 39, 42, 43, 44, 46, 49, 54, 61, 69
differential diagnosis, 37, 53
digestion, 10, 39
dilated cardiomyopathy, 45
diseases, 3, 10, 16, 21, 24, 26, 31, 35, 50, 60, 61, 70
disequilibrium, 27
disorder, 1, 2, 22, 42, 50, 60
distribution, 7, 27
donors, 23
dosage, 9, 57, 58, 60, 62, 69, 70
dosing, 74
Down syndrome, 8, 16, 62
drug-resistant epilepsy, 20
drugs, 20
duodenum, 33, 37
dyspepsia, 16

E

edema, 2, 12
Egypt, 3
elbows, 23
electrolyte imbalance, 13
enamel, 13
encephalopathy, 20
encoding, 2, 9
endocardium, 22
endocrine, 8, 50, 53
endocrine disorders, 8
endocrinology, 71
endoscopy, 32
enteritis, 36, 37
enteropathy, 3, 4, 11, 12, 13, 15, 16, 21, 23, 30, 37, 46
environmental factors, 1, 8, 9, 27
enzymatic activity, 30
enzyme, 6, 10, 30, 31, 39
enzyme immunoassay, 6
enzyme-linked immunosorbent assay, 31
enzymes, 26
epidemiology, 1, 7
epilepsy, 20, 45
epithelial cells, 30, 33
epithelium, 11, 35
epitopes, 8, 10, 21, 28, 39
equilibrium, 40
esophagus, 16, 18, 31
etiology, 36
Europe, vii, 1, 6
everyday life, 3
evidence, 10, 13, 20, 21, 24, 27, 36, 41, 42, 61, 70
evolution, 6, 23, 26
examinations, 62
exclusion, 49, 53, 73
execution, 69
exercise, 41, 74
exposure, 3, 11, 21, 27, 46, 60
extensor, 23
extracellular matrix, 30

F

failure to thrive, 13, 16
false positive, 31, 35
family members, 29, 38, 42
family physician, 18
fat, 69
fibroblasts, 10
fibrogenesis, 27
fibrosis, 24, 25
fibrous tissue, 36
Finland, 6, 27
flatulence, 16
flour, 4, 41
fluctuations, 72
fluorescence, 19, 31
folate, 17, 20
folic acid, 13
food, 3, 36, 39, 41, 42
force, 5
formation, 22
formula, 64
fractures, 19

G

gait, 21
gastritis, 17
gastrointestinal tract, 16, 18
general practitioner, 18, 32
genes, 2, 8, 9
genetic background, 21
genetic disorders, 8
genetic marker, 27
genetic predisposition, 1, 2, 8, 9, 27, 38
genetics, 46
genome, 8
genotype, 32
Germany, 6
gland, 51, 55
glial cells, 20
glucagon, 68, 72
glucose, 55, 62, 69, 71, 72
glucose tolerance, 55, 62

glutamine, 10, 30, 40
glycoproteins, 8
growth, 2, 12, 16, 17, 22, 43, 49, 50, 51, 52, 53, 54, 55, 57, 59, 61, 62, 63, 64, 65, 66, 69, 70, 72, 75
growth factor, 54
growth hormone, 16, 50, 72, 75
growth rate, 49, 52, 54, 58, 63, 73
guidelines, vii, 5, 29, 33, 44, 68, 73, 75

H

hair, 65
haplotypes, 8, 9, 27
health, 23, 39
health care, 39
heart disease, 17
height, vii, 33, 49, 51, 52, 53, 55, 58, 59, 63, 64, 65, 69, 76
Helicobacter pylori, 35, 36
hematology, 18
hemoglobin, 69, 70
hepatic failure, 27, 46
hepatitis, 17, 24, 25, 26, 27, 29, 46, 47
hepatitis a, 25
hepatitis d, 26
hepatocellular carcinoma, 24
herpes virus, 37
histocompatibility class, 1, 8
histology, 25, 36, 47
HLA, 1, 5, 6, 8, 9, 10, 21, 22, 27, 28, 29, 32, 37, 38, 43, 44, 60
hormone, 16, 50, 58, 69, 70, 71, 72, 75, 76
hormones, 55, 56, 62
Hospital for Sick Children, 3
host, 37
human, 2, 6, 28, 29, 31, 40, 55
human condition, 2
hydrocortisone, 57, 58
hyperparathyroidism, 17, 19
hyperplasia, 5, 11, 24, 25, 33, 34
hypersensitivity, 35, 36, 41
hypertension, 70
hypoglycemia, 71
hypotension, 13, 41

hypothalamus, 62
hypothyroidism, 53, 73

I

iatrogenic, 20
identification, 39, 41
idiopathic, 20, 22, 36, 45, 50, 55, 57, 58, 59, 61
imbalances, 13
immune response, 8, 9, 28
immunity, 40
immunocompetent cells, 8
immunodeficiency, 36
immunofluorescence, 19, 23, 35
immunoglobulin, 28, 29, 30, 32
immunohistochemistry, 15
immunomodulation, 39
immunostimulatory, 10
incidence, 8, 27, 70
individuals, 6, 8, 9, 11, 19, 21, 25, 27, 32, 39, 40, 60
INF, 10
infants, 22, 41
infection, 30, 37
infertility, 22
inflammation, 25, 27
inflammatory bowel disease, 36
inflammatory cells, 10
ingestion, 2, 39, 41, 42
inhibition, 40
inhibitor, 40
initiation, 49, 54
injury, 46
inoculation, 69
insulin, 61, 68, 69, 70, 71, 72
insulin resistance, 70
interferon, 60
interferon-γ, 60
intestinal malabsorption, 53
intestinal mucosa, 4, 6, 9, 10, 11, 15, 16, 18, 28, 30, 36, 38, 61
intestine, 4, 6, 8, 11, 24, 40
intolerance to gluten, 11
intravenously, 68, 71, 72

iron, 13, 14, 16, 17, 18, 44
irradiation, 68
irritability, 13
irritable bowel syndrome, 13, 42
Italy, 1, 7, 18, 49

J

jejunum, 30
joints, 27

K

karyotype, 62
kidney, 53

L

lactose intolerance, 19
lamina propria, 10, 11, 30
latency, 11, 30
lead, 20, 39
lesions, 11, 23, 24, 32, 33, 34, 46
lethargy, 13, 41
leukemia, 70
liver, 16, 17, 24, 25, 26, 27, 28, 46, 53
liver damage, 24, 25, 27
liver disease, 16, 24, 25, 26, 27, 28, 46, 53
liver enzymes, 26
liver function tests, 25
liver transplantation, 27
lumen, 28
lupus, 35
lymphocytes, 6, 9, 10, 11, 15, 21, 33, 34, 35, 36
lymphocytosis, 33, 36
lymphoid, 36, 40
lymphoid tissue, 40
lymphoma, 15, 16, 18, 37
lysine, 30

M

macromolecules, 40, 60
magnetic resonance, 21, 55, 62
magnetic resonance imaging, 21, 55
malabsorption, 12, 13, 16, 17, 19, 20, 42, 50, 53
malignancy, 39
malnutrition, 2, 12, 50, 58, 73
management, 41, 47
mass, 38, 64, 69, 70
mass loss, 70
matrix, 10, 30
matrix metalloproteinase, 10
measurements, 62, 63, 68, 75
mechanical stress, 30
medical, 32, 43
medical history, 43
Mediterranean countries, 39
medulla, 21
mellitus, 8, 50, 60, 70
menarche, 22, 66
menopause, 22
mental retardation, 20
methodology, 68
Middle East, 6
mineralization, 19
miscarriages, 22
mitosis, 33
modifications, 10
molecules, 1, 6, 8, 9, 10, 27
monozygotic twins, 8
morbidity, 23
morphology, 4, 11, 65
mortality, 3, 39
mortality risk, 3
mucosa, 4, 6, 9, 10, 11, 15, 16, 18, 28, 30, 35, 36
mucosal sensitivity, 4
multipotent, 39
muscles, 27
myocardium, 22
myoclonus, 21
myopathy, 17
myosin, 22

N

nausea, 72
negativity, 55
nervous system, 27, 68
Netherlands, 4
neuroimaging, 20
neurological disease, 20
neurons, 20
neuropathy, 21
New Zealand, 6
normal children, 55
normal development, 66
North Africa, 6
North America, vii, viii, 74
nuclear magnetic resonance, 55
nutrients, 24
nutrition, 23
nutritional status, 54, 56

O

occupational asthma, 41
oral cavity, 16, 18
organ(s), 21, 24, 27, 62
osteoporosis, 14, 19, 45
outpatient, 18
overweight, 64, 69

P

pain, 13, 16, 17, 42
pallor, 41
pancreas, 27
parenchyma, 60
parents, 38, 69
paresthesias, 70
pathogenesis, 19, 21, 27, 30, 50
pathologist, 35
pathology, 53, 68
PCR, 15
pediatrician, 3, 63
peptidase, 40
peptides, 5, 8, 9, 10, 21, 31, 39, 40, 73
peripheral neuropathy, 21
permeability, 10, 28, 39, 40, 50, 60
phagocytosis, 30
pharynx, 16, 18
phenotype, 15, 74
physicians, vii, 18
placebo, 40, 42
polymerization, 10
pons, 21
population, 1, 6, 9, 15, 17, 18, 19, 20, 21, 22, 23, 26, 31, 35, 36, 38, 41, 42, 45, 46, 47, 60, 63
population growth, 63
pregnancy, 23, 45
primary biliary cirrhosis, 26
priming, 62, 68, 73
prognosis, 20
pro-inflammatory, 9
proline, 39
proteins, 2, 5, 12, 30, 39
pubertal development, 62, 64, 70, 73
puberty, 13, 14, 50, 52, 55, 66, 68, 69, 70, 73

Q

quality of life, 13

R

radiation, 37
rash, 70
reactions, 42, 70
reactivity, 21, 30
receptors, 71
recognition, 9, 10, 41
recommendations, 33, 74
recurrence, 4
reintroduction, 4, 41
relapses, 28
relatives, 8, 9, 31, 38
remission, 2, 5, 28
repair, 38

Index

resistance, 70
resolution, 38, 55
response, 2, 4, 5, 6, 8, 9, 11, 15, 21, 23, 28, 40, 44, 47, 55, 57, 59, 62, 69, 70, 71, 72, 74
restoration, 28
retardation, 20
RH, 75
rheumatoid arthritis, 35, 36
rhinitis, 41
risk, 3, 9, 10, 13, 15, 16, 18, 19, 20, 22, 23, 26, 27, 38, 39, 44, 45, 46, 60, 61, 70, 73
rotavirus, 10
rubella, 23

S

safety, 39, 40
scoliosis, 70
secrete, 10, 72
secretion, 49, 54, 55, 57, 61, 62, 68, 70, 71, 72, 73
sensitivity, 2, 4, 12, 31, 32, 41, 43, 48, 55, 70, 73
sensitization, 20, 41
sepsis, 19, 45
serologic test, 30
serology, 11, 15, 39, 43, 55, 61
serum, 11, 30, 31, 38, 42, 46, 72, 73
sex, 50, 55, 68, 73
sex steroid, 68, 73
showing, 20, 66, 73
side effects, 40, 70, 72, 73
signs, 2, 3, 11, 12, 13, 15, 20, 21, 25, 32, 38, 42, 51, 55
single test, 31
skin, 23, 27, 41, 46, 70
small intestine, 4, 8, 11, 24, 40
smooth muscle, 31
sodium, 70
South America, 6
soybeans, 35
sprue, 36, 37
stabilization, 30
standard deviation, 55, 57, 58, 62

steatorrhea, 2, 12
steroids, 68, 73
stimulation, 68, 71, 73
stimulus, 55, 58, 62, 68, 72
stomatitis, 13, 14, 17
stress, 30
structure, 24, 31, 60
subgroups, 34
submucosa, 6, 8
substitutes (substitution), 40
substrate, 31
supplementation, 14
surface component, 31
surveillance, 71
susceptibility, 1, 8, 11, 38
symptoms, 1, 2, 3, 5, 7, 11, 12, 13, 15, 16, 19, 21, 22, 23, 25, 32, 38, 40, 41, 42, 43, 50, 75
syndrome, 2, 8, 12, 13, 16, 17, 20, 24, 37, 38, 41, 42, 62, 70, 74
systemic lupus erythematosus, 35

T

T lymphocytes, 6, 9, 10, 11, 15, 21, 33, 35, 36
target, 30, 39, 51, 62, 64
T-cell receptor, 15
techniques, 7, 35
technologies, 39
testing, 2, 13, 29, 30, 31, 32, 37, 38, 43
testosterone, 57, 68, 73
therapy, 18, 28, 39, 50, 55, 57, 58, 59, 61, 62, 69, 70, 74, 76
thrombocytosis, 18
thyroglobulin, 60
thyroid, 16, 17, 27, 50, 56, 58, 60, 61, 62, 69
thyroiditis, 8, 35, 36, 60
tissue, 6, 10, 19, 28, 29, 30, 31, 32, 35, 36, 40, 50, 61
TNF-α, 60
total cholesterol, 69
toxicity, 39
toxoplasmosis, 23

transaminases, 25
transplantation, 27
trauma, 23
treatment, vii, 38, 39, 40, 47, 55, 56, 57, 58, 59, 60, 62, 69, 70, 74, 75
triggers, 23
TSH, 55, 56, 58, 60, 62, 69
tuberculosis, 37
tumors, 70
twins, 8
type 1 diabetes, 45, 60
type 2 diabetes, 70

U

umbilical cord, 31
urticaria, 41
USA, 76

V

vaccine, 39

valuation, 53, 68, 70
variables, 69
velocity, 58, 59, 62, 63, 64, 65, 70
vessels, 21
villus, 34, 35, 36
viral infection, 30
vitamin D, 19
vomiting, 41, 72

W

water, 70
weight loss, 12, 13, 16
withdrawal, 4, 5, 24, 25, 26, 28

Z

zinc, 50, 61